T0187551

COMPUTATIONAL MODELLING AND IMAGING FOR SARS-COV-2 AND COVID-19

COMPUTATIONAL MODELLING AND IMAGING FOR SARS-COV-2 AND COVID-19

Edited by
S. Prabha, P. Karthikeyan, K. Kamalanand, and
N. Selvaganesan

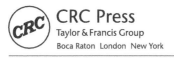

CRC Press
Taylor & Francis Group
Boca Raton   London   New York

CRC Press is an imprint of the
Taylor & Francis Group, an **informa** business

First edition published 2022
by CRC Press
2 Park Square, Milton Park, Abingdon, Oxon, OX14 4RN

and by CRC Press
6000 Broken Sound Parkway NW, Suite 300, Boca Raton, FL 33487-2742

British Library Cataloguing-in-Publication Data
A catalogue record for this book is available from the British Library

Library of Congress Cataloging-in-Publication Data
Names: Prabha, S., editor. | Karthikeyan, P., Dr., editor. | Kamalanand, K., 1988- editor. |
Selvaganesan, N., editor.
Title: Computational modelling and imaging for SARS-CoV-2 and COVID-19 / edited by S.
Prabha, P. Karthikeyan, K. Kamalanand, N. Selvaganesan. Description: First edition. | Boca
Raton : CRC Press, 2022. | Includes bibliographical references and index. |
Summary: "This book presents new computational techniques and methodologies for the
analysis of the clinical, epidemiological and public health aspects of SARS-CoV-2 and
COVID-19 pandemic. The book presents the use of soft computing techniques such as
machine learning algorithms for analysis of the epidemiological aspects of the SARS-CoV-
2"-- Provided by publisher.
Identifiers: LCCN 2021013495 (print) | LCCN 2021013496 (ebook) | ISBN 9780367695293
(hardback) | ISBN 9780367696245 (paperback) | ISBN 9781003142584 (ebook)
Subjects: MESH: COVID-19--diagnostic imaging | Radiographic Image Interpretation,
Computer-Assisted--methods | COVID-19--epidemiology | SARS-CoV-2 | Computer
Simulation | Models, Statistical | Artificial Intelligence
Classification: LCC RA644.C67 (print) | LCC RA644.C67 (ebook) | NLM WC 506.1 | DDC
616.2/414075--dc23
LC record available at https://lccn.loc.gov/2021013495
LC ebook record available at https://lccn.loc.gov/2021013496

ISBN: 978-0-367-69529-3 (hbk)
ISBN: 978-0-367-69624-5 (pbk)
ISBN: 978-1-003-14258-4 (ebk)

Typeset in Times
by MPS Limited, Dehradun

Contents

Preface

SARS-CoV-2 is a highly contagious RNA virus that was first identified in Wuhan, China. As of 8th March 2021, the COVID-19 epidemic has affected 219 countries worldwide, with a total of 117,446,648 infected individuals and 2,605,302 reported deaths throughout the globe. The World Health Organization (WHO) has declared COVID-19 a pandemic and at present several countries are going through a second wave. Since COVID-19 infection leads to symptoms ranging from mild to severe, and the transmission rate (R0) of the epidemic ranges from 1.5 to 3.5, this infection has a high impact on public health. Further, the incubation period of COVID-19 infection falls between 2 to 14 days, during which the SARS-CoV-2 is contagious, but the infected individuals do not display any symptoms. Hence, it is highly important to offer timely research and information of various aspects of SARS-CoV-2 and the COVID-19 epidemic. This edited book is an effort to highlight the computational and mathematical tools for computer-assisted analysis of the SARS-CoV-2 infection. This book entitled "Computational Modelling and Imaging for SARS-CoV-2 and COVID-19" covers a variety of topics on the imaging aspects of COVID-19 detection and staging of the infection, and progression modelling of the epidemic using machine learning and analyzing the effect of interventions on the epidemic.

This book is organized into eight chapters. The first chapter, entitled "Artificial-Intelligence-Based COVID-19 Detection using Medical-Imaging Methods: A Review", authored by Murugappan et al., provides a general introduction to the COVID-19 epidemic and offers several artificial-intelligence-based schemes for detection using radiographic images. The second chapter, entitled "Review of Imaging Features for COVID-19", authored by Chitradevi and Prabha, presents a review of imaging features of different modalities, namely, Radiography, Positron Tomography, Ultrasonography, Magnetic Resonance Imaging and Computed Tomography, and their application in analysis of the SARS-CoV-2 infection. The third chapter, entitled "Investigation of COVID-19 Chest X-ray Images Using Texture Features – A Comprehensive approach", authored by Thamil Selvi et al., presents an attempt to investigate normal and COVID-19-positive chest X-ray images using texture features. The fourth chapter, entitled "Efficient Diagnosis using Chest CT in COVID-19: A Review", authored by Sivakama-sundari and Venkatesh, offers a review of the techniques for analysis of COVID-19 infection in chest CT images, since they offer a better tool for analysing the complications of COVID-19 infection.

Since it is well established that the use of surgical masks and N95 masks can slow down the transmission of the COVID-19 epidemic, the fifth chapter, entitled "Automatic Mask Detection and Social Distance Alerting Based on a Deep- Learning Computer-Vision Algorithm", authored by Vinoth et al., presents an approach based on a deep-learning algorithm to detect people with and without a mask, along with the social distancing protocol in public places.

The sixth chapter, entitled "Review of Effective Mathematical Modelling of Corona-virus Epidemic and the Effect of Drone Disinfection", authored by Jayaprakash et al., analyses the effect of intervention strategies on the COVID-19 epidemic using a mathematical-modelling approach. The seventh chapter, entitled "ANFIS Algorithm-Based Modeling and Forecasting of the COVID-19 Epidemic: A Case Study in Tamil Nadu, India", authored by Vijayakarthick et al., presents an ANFIS model for predicting the progression of the epidemic in terms of both active cases and deaths. The final chapter, entitled "Prediction and Analysis of SARS-CoV-2 (COVID-19) Epidemic in India using an LSTM Network", authored by Ganesh Ram et al., proposes an LSTM network and moving average technique for predicting the confirmed, active and deceased cases in India.

This book aims to offer timely literature on computational/imaging aspects of the SARS-CoV-2 infection. We thank Dr. Marc Gutierrez, Editor, and Dr. Nick Mould, Editorial Assistant, CRC press, for their continuous support from the initial stage to final publication. We hope that this book is interesting and informative to its users.

S. Prabha
P. Karthikeyan
K. Kamalanand
N. Selvaganesan

Editors

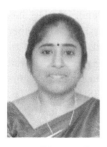

Dr. S. Prabha completed her Ph.D. degree at the College of Engineering, Guindy Campus, Anna University, in the field of "Analysis of Breast Thermograms using Adaptive Level Set and Riesz Transform". Currently, she is working as an associate professor in the Department of Electronics and Communication Engineering, Hindustan Institute of Technology and Science, Chennai, India. Her research interests include image and signal processing, biomedical instrumentation, biometric security and cloud computing. She has published in many edited Books, reputed international journals and conferences. She has secured two best paper awards and is a member of IEEE, IET and ISOI.

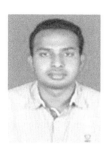

Dr. P. Karthikeyan received an M.E. (Mechatronics) First Class with Distinction at the Madras Institute of Technology, Anna University, India. He has completed his Ph.D. (Mechatronic Engineering) at the School of Mechatronics Engineering, Universiti Malaysia Perlis (UniMAP), Malaysia, in the area of signal processing and information fusion. He is currently working as an assistant professor in the Department of Production Technology, Madras Institute of Technology, Anna University, India. Additionally, he is deputy director of the Centre for Academic Courses, Anna University, Chennai. His teaching and research interest include mechatronic system design and modelling, as well as control, signal and information processing for decision making in intelligent automation.

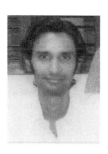

Dr. K. Kamalanand completed his Ph.D. at the MIT Campus, Anna University, in the field of "HIV/AIDS modelling". At present he is an assistant professor in the Department of Instrumentation Engineering, Madras Institute of Technology Campus, Anna University, Chennai, India. He is well-published, with five books, nine chapters in edited books, 37 research articles in international journals, and 20 articles in conference proceedings. He has served as a guest editor for the *European Journal for Biomedical Informatics* (Official journal of the European Federation for Medical Informatics), and *Current Bioinformatics, Current Signal Transduction Therapy* (Bentham Science). He is a member of the Council of Asian Science Editors, and the International Society of Infectious Diseases.

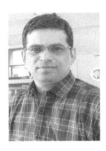 **Dr. N. Selvaganesan** received his Ph.D. in Adaptive Control Systems from the MIT Campus, Anna University, Chennai in the year 2005. He has more than 19 years of research and teaching experience. Currently, he is working as a professor in the Department of Avionics in IIST-Trivandrum. He has served in many administrative positions at IIST and other institutions/universities, which include Head, Department of Avionics, IIST during 2013–16. He has 33 peer- reviewed international journal papers and 42 conference papers to his research credit. He has completed research projects sponsored by ISRO and DSTE. His current research direction is towards human health monitoring and fault diagnosis of crew module/flight control in space. He is involved in many editorial activities and reviews for various international journals, conferences and workshops (Control System Design-CSD). His areas of interest include control system design, estimation theory, biological modelling, fault diagnosis and fractional order control. He is a senior member of IEEE.

Contributors

Ali K. Bourisly
Department of Physiology Faculty of Medicine Kuwait University Doha
Doha, Kuwait

D. Chitradevi
Department of CSE, Hindustan Institute of Technology and Science
Chennai, India

Agnishwar Jayaprakash
Agni Foundation
Chennai, India

Palani Thanaraj Krishnan
Department of Electronics and Instrumentation Engineering, St. Joseph's College of Engineering, Anna University
Chennai, India

Vasanthan Maruthapillai
Faculty of Engineering and Information Technology, Southern University College
Johor Bharu, Malaysia

M. Methini
Department of ECE, Sri Sairam Engineering College
Chennai, India

S. Meyyappan
Department of Instrumentation Engineering, Madras Institute of Technology Campus, Anna University
Chennai, India

Hariharan Muthusamy
Department of Electronics Engineering National Institute of Technology Srinagar (Garhwal)
Uttarakhand, India

M. Murugappan
Department of Electronics and Communication Engineering, Kuwait College of Science and Technology (A Private University), Block 4
Doha, Kuwait

R. Nithya
Department of Biomedical Engineering, Agni college of Technology
Chennai, India

S. Prabha
Department of ECE, Hindustan Institute of Technology and Science
Chennai, India

J. Thamil Selvi
Department of ECE, Sri Sairam Engineering College
Chennai, India

J. Sivakamasundari
Department of Biomedical Engineering, Jerusalem College of Engineering
Chennai, India

E. Sivaraman
Department of Electronics and Communication Engineering, GCE
Tirunelveli, India

K. Subhashini
Department of ECE, Sri Sairam
    Engineering College
Chennai, India

K. Venkatesh
Kovai Medical Center and Hospital
    Coimbatore
Tamil Nadu, India

M. Vijayakarthick
Department of Instrumentation
    Engineering, Madras Institute of
    Technology Campus, Anna
    University
Chennai, India

N. Vinoth
Department of Instrumentation
    Engineering, Madras Institute of
    Technology Campus, Anna
    University
Chennai, India

A. Ganesh Ram
Department of Instrumentation
    Engineering, Madras Institute of
    Technology Campus, Anna
    University
Chennai, India

1 Artificial Intelligence Based COVID-19 Detection using Medical Imaging Methods: A Review

M Murugappan[1], Ali K Bourisly[2], Palani Thanaraj Krishnan[3], Vasanthan Maruthapillai[4], and Hariharan Muthusamy[5]*

[1]Department of Electronics and Communication Engineering, Kuwait College of Science and Technology (A Private University), Block 4, Doha, Kuwait
[2]Department of Physiology, Faculty of Medicine, Kuwait University, Kuwait
[3]Department of Electronics and Instrumentation Engineering, St. Joseph's College of Engineering, Anna University, Chennai, India
[4]Faculty of Engineering and Information Technology, Southern University College, Johor Bharu, Malaysia
[5]Department of Electronics Engineering, National Institute of Technology, Srinagar (Garhwal), Uttarakhand, India
[*]Corresponding Author Email: m.murugappan@gmail.com, m.murugappan@kcst.edu.kw

1.1 INTRODUCTION

The novel coronavirus was first found in Wuhan, China, on Dec 2019, and was spread over 218 countries/territories by 26 October 2020, with nearly 43 million people infected and around 1 million deaths worldwide (Europa Data 2020). Now, the novel coronavirus infection is officially referred to as COVID-19 disease. The coronavirus that causes this disease is the Severe Acute Respiratory Syndrome (SARS-CoV-2), an RNA-type virus which is a challenge to the scientific community as it is difficult to characterize. COVID-19 is a deadly virus. It enters the human body through droplets and close contact, starts changing its genetic code and

1

rapidly spreads among organs, specifically the lungs, over a short period. Some of the most challenging factors behind COVID-19 are: (i) it does not have any standard genetic code to describe its behaviour; (ii) symptoms of this virus differ from person to person based on their antibody behaviour; and (iii) symptoms and effects of this virus are not always immmediatly apparent. Because of the above characteristics, vaccine development for COVID-19 is more challenging. Researchers are developing several vaccines for testing. Furthermore, this virus spreads among humans through respiratory droplets and close contact; it stays alive in the air for more than 3 hours. COVID-19 is a lower-respiratory-tract infection which is different from the common cold, an upper-respiratory-tract infection. Moreover, COVID-19 can cause severe breathing problems and pneumonia.

1.1.1 STATISTICS

The World Health Organization (WHO) declared the COVID-19 a pandemic disease in February 2020 (another name for COVID-19 is Severe Acute Respiratory Syndrome coronavirus-2 or SARS – CoV-2) (WHO-Coronavirus 2020, Stoecklin et al. 2020). There are 218 countries/regions affected by COVID-19. According to recent statistics from Johns Hopkins University (JHU), there are 43,009,98 confirmed cases in the world and total mortalities due to COVID-19 increased to 1,153,861 as of 26 October 2020 (Europa Data 2020, Corona eGov Kuwait COVID-19 Updates 2020, COVID-19 Alibabacloud 2020). A statistical report states that nearly 95%of infected patients survive the disease, while 5% become seriously or critically ill (NGC-Coronavirus 2020). Countries like the USA, India, Brazil, Russia and Argentina have the most confirmed cases of COVID-19. Table 1.1 reports the top 5 worst-affected countries by number of confirmed cases, new cases and death reported in the last 24 hours and total deaths (NIH harnesses AI 2020).

TABLE 1.1
Top 5 worst-affected countries due to COVID-19*

Country	Confirmed Cases	Cases Newly Reported in Last 24 hr	Deaths Newly Reported in Last 24 hr	Total Deaths	Transmission Classification
USA	8,403,121	82,630	943	222,507	Community
India	7,864,811	50,129	578	118,534	Cluster of cases
Brazil	5,353,656	30,026	571	156,471	Community
Russia	1,513,877	16,710	229	26,050	Cluster of cases
Argentina	1,069,368	15,718	381	28,338	Community transmission

Notes:
* https://covid19.who.int/ [Accessed on 26/10/2020]

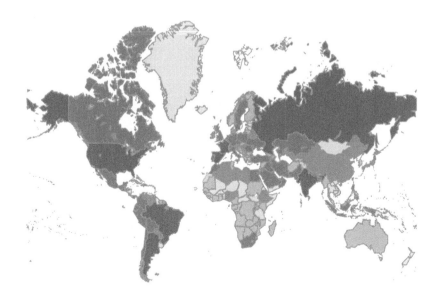

FIGURE 1.1   Choropleth map of the world (total number of confirmed cases of COVID-19).

Figure 1.1 shows the choropleth map of the world (confirmed cases of COVID-19 and total deaths) accessed on 26 October 2020. From Figure 1.1, it is observed how the novel coronavirus is spreading around the globe; more than 218 countries or regions are affected by the deadly novel coronavirus (WHO Coronavirus Dashboard 2020). The USA, India, Brazil, Russia and Argentina have the most confirmed cases of COVID-19, represented in Figure.1.1 in dark blue. From Figure 1.2, it can be noted that the rapid spread of COVID-19 virus has resulted in a massive increase of deaths. A maximum number of deaths has been reported in the USA, Brazil, Argentina, Spain, the UK, Italy, Mexico and France due to COVID-19.

1.1.2 Clinical Symptoms, Manifestations and their Effects

The COVID-19 virus has symptoms similar to other coronaviruses, such as Severe Acute Respiratory Syndrome (SARS) and Middle East Respiratory Syndrome (MERS) (WHO-Coronavirus 2020, Huang et al. 2020, Chowdary et al. 2020). Current clinical manifestations of COVID-19 can include: (i) fever; (ii) breathing trouble; (iii) pneumonia; (iv) reduced white blood cell count (WBC); (vi) rapid increase in erythrocyte sedimentation rate (ESR); and (vii) reduced lymphocyte count. Clinical symptoms of COVID-19 have been classified into four different stages: mild; moderate; severe; and critical (Worldmeters-Coronavirus 2020). According to a recent study, most COVID-19 patients have mild symptoms. The signs of a mild infection include fever, cough, dyspnea, respiratory symptoms (i.e., breathing difficulties or short breath), muscle ache, diarrhoea, and headache (WHO-Coronavirus 2020). The signs of moderate infection include high fever and

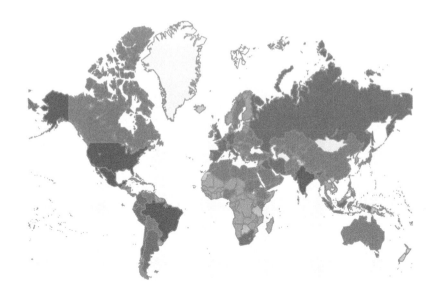

FIGURE 1.2   Choropleth map of the world (total number of deaths of COVID-19).

pneumonia symptoms. Respiratory distress (Respiration rate ≥ 30 times/min) and oxygen saturation ≤ 93% in a resting state are the most common signs of severe infection. However, respiratory failure, septic shock, multi-organ failure, Severe Acute Respiratory Syndrome (SARS), and death are signs of the critical stage (Mahase 2020, Wang et al. 2020b).

The most common effects of COVID-19 are respiratory problems due to viral infection of the lungs. This virus goes inside the human body through the oral pathway, and starts changing its genetic code over the infection's duration. It then creates ground-glass opacities (GGO), multiple ground-glass opacities (MGGO), and lesions, which infiltrate the lungs, and enlarge the lymph nodes (Guardian:COVID-19 2020, Itnonline:COVID-19 2020, European Lung 2020). The effects of COVID-19 are quite similar to other viruses, such as SARS and MERS, and it is highly challenging to differentiate pneumonia due to COVID-19. According to a recent report of researchers from China, those with A + blood and those older than 55 are profoundly affected by COVID-19 over the world. Besides, patients with a history of chronic disease are more easily affected by COVID-19, compared to healthy individuals.

1.2   DIAGNOSIS METHODS AND NEED FOR AN AI-BASED SOLUTION

Currently, COVID-19 has been conclusively diagnosed through molecular tests ((polymerase chain reaction (PCR) and real-time reverse transcription-polymerase chain reaction test (RT-PCR)) with a high success rate. However, due to limited facilities to perform molecular or rapid antigen tests (RAT), most countries require more than 48 hours to disclose results of the COVID-19 diagnosis. The present clinical procedure to detect COVID-19 is minimally invasive at best, but requires more facilities, trained human resources (epidemiologist or virologist), and time.

Diagnosis of COVID-19 relies on the following criteria: (a) clinical symptoms; (b) clinical imaging (i.e., Computed Tomography (CT) and general X-Ray images); (c) nucleic acid test/pathogenic testing; (d) close contact history; (e) contact history with patients with fever; (f) clustering occurrence; and (g) epidemiological history (Sana et al. 2020, Radiology assistant 2020). The standard test recommended by the WHO to diagnose COVID-19 is the Nucleic Acid Amplification Test (NAAT) and RT-PCR (Hao & Li 2020, EUA-COVID-19 2020). Sudden increase in levels of C-reactive protein and ESR is used as an additional tool for diagnosing COVID-19. Significant limitations of RT-PCR testing are: (a) many countries do not have abundant access to sophisticated labs and appropriate laboratory tools to perform this test; (b) the test is supposed to be repeated 2 to 3 times to validate the accuracy of results; (c) limited access to virologists and epidemiologists in many countries slows down the diagnosis process; (d) turnaround time to get the results of RT-PCR can be up to 72 hours for one sample; (e) testing is expensive and could not be afforded by developing countries; and (f) finally, it is minimally invasive (Soon et al. 2020). The above limitations of RT-PCR are also valid for the NAAT test; however, if the viral load is low while testing, the NAAT test results will be negative (Ying et al. 2020). All the above issues significantly delay the diagnosis process. Early isolation stops the spread and allows treatment to start early.

Because of the limitations of RT-PCR and NAAT mentioned above, clinical imaging methods also play a vital role in diagnosis in countries where conventional methods are inaccessible. As of early Feb 2020, many countries do not have the facilities to perform RT-PCR tests utilizing radio-imaging methods as first-line tools to diagnose COVID-19. Some of the most common clinical imaging tools used for COVID-19 diagnosis are ultrasound images, chest Computed Tomography (CT) scanning, and chest X-Ray (). These imaging methods are mostly found in hospitals, they are affordable, give accurate results as compared to RT-PCT in a short period. They also offer faster response time and are non-invasive. X-Ray images are mostly used for clinical diagnoses such as bone fractures, bone relocation, tumour identification, lung infections, and pneumonia. In the case of X-Ray imaging, the significant advantages are that it is convenient, economic and available in all hospitals and clinics. Several research works have used chest x-ray (CXR) images to develop an intelligent COVID-19 diagnosis system using AI methods (Feng et al. 2020, Ozturk et al. 2020, Abbas et al. 2020, Khan et al. 2020, Sethy et al. 2020, Mukherjee et al. 2020, Ucar et al. 2020, Kumar et al. 2020, Afshar et al. 2020, Farooq et al. 2020, Basu et al. 2020, Chowdhury et al. 2020, Li et al. 2020a, Narin et al. 2020, Mahdy et al. 2020). However, X-Ray images are not suitable for analyzing ground-glass opacities, crazy paving patterns, or multiple ground-glass opacities due to its low image resolution. The above indications are more prevalent in COVID-19 pneumonia compared to other viral pneumonia. Hence, significant preprocessing methods are required to improve image contrast for better clinical diagnosis. Compared to X-Ray images, a CT scan is mostly used for investigating the soft structure of the active body, and it gives clear, high-resolution images of soft tissues and organs (Li et al. 2020, Ho et al. 2020). Hence, most of the earlier works and physicians preferred to use CT scan images compared to X-Ray images in the clinical diagnosis of COVID-19 (Wei-cai et al. 2020, Shuai et al. 2020, Ran et al. 2020, Lu et al. 2020, Ophir et al. 2020, Lin et al. 2020, Wang et al. 2020, Singh et al. 2020, Abdullah et al. 2020, Li et al. 2020, Xu et al. 2020, Chen et al. 2020, Elghamrawy et al. 2020, Shan et al. 2020, He et al. 2020, Amyar et al. 2020). Collective findings from chest CT scan images are categorized into five different stages in COVID-19 detection: (i) Ultra-early (No pneumonia symptoms, CT scan images may show single or multiple GGO, air bronchogram after 1-2 weeks of infection); (ii) Early (single or multiple GGO and interlobar septal thickening); (iii) Rapid progression (large, light consolidative opacities, and air bronchogram); (iv) Consolidation (reduction in density and size of consolidative opacities); and finally (v) Dissipation, with death resulting from organ failure (Ran et al. 2020). This classification is performed by investigating the morphological features of GGO and lesions, such as size, density, area, depth, and location in the lung region. It is also important to note that access to CT imaging may be a challenge compared to RT-PCR and NAAT, as it requires patients to enter a hospital, and these imaging modalities are also limited. It is more challenging to deploy on mobile bases. Hence, most investigators are interested in carrying out an investigative study to develop an intelligent COVID-19 diagnosis system to aid in classification of COVID-19 patients. This is done by observing respiratory symptoms, which may go unnoticed by fatigued radiologists. It also helps in automation so that clinicians can free up time to focus on other clinical issues and administration during COVID-19.

To circumvent these issues of conventional COVID-19 detection methods, researchers started developing artificial-intelligence-based clinical diagnosis systems for speeding up the early detection of COVID-19. Perhaps imaging could aid in screening or accelerate the speed of diagnosis, especially with shortages of RT-PCR. Hence, most of the recent works in the literature aim to design and develop an AI-based algorithm using medical-imaging methods to detect COVID-19 in such a way to help doctors to diagnose COVID-19 patients. This will also help them decide what to do next, depending on the output of the algorithm, help automate the diagnosis/prognosis of COVID-19 patients to help doctors determine the severity of COVID-19 and tell them how to proceed for patients. Consequently, doctors' time will be saved as the algorithm will automate a process that can be very time-consuming.

1.3   ARTIFICIAL INTELLIGENCE METHODS

Artificial-Intelligence-based (AI-based) clinical diagnosis systems are prevalent in many healthcare systems; they have resulted in paradigm shifts over recent years in healthcare delivery. The power of AI-based systems is that they produce accurate and reliable diagnosis results in a short period without fatigue. Also, AI systems are used to improve the workflow of a healthcare system by reducing the burden on human resources. In the case of COVID-19 detection, AI systems have been used to detect lesions and ground-glass opacities (GGO) in the CT scan images, which is faster compared to a manual clinical specialist diagnosis, thereby saving time of clinical specialists/physicians and significantly aiding them in the sometimes lengthy process of manually reading images one by one to identify high-risk cases. It also may significantly reduce patient time in the hospital, which poses a severe risk of spreading the virus (McCall 2020, Ali et al. 2020). Figure 1.2 illustrates the methodologies developed for the diagnosis of COVID infection from radiographic images (CT/X-ray) using various machine-learning and deep- learning methods (Figure 1.3).

Extracting COVID-19-related features from chest CT scan is highly complex, challenging, and time-consuming; a simple calculation may not work well with the CT scan image data and needs many repetitions for decision making. Therefore, machine-learning methods have been applied to COVID-19 detection using chest CT scan images (Shuai et al. 2020, Lu et al. 2020, Ophir et al. 2020, Lin et al. 2020). Machine learning is a branch of artificial intelligence based on the idea that systems can learn from data, identify patterns, and make decisions with minimal human intervention; this method automates analytical model building. Machine learning has been used as a decision-making algorithm for unknown chest CT scan images based on a set of training data, and past studies have implemented machine learning on COVID-19 detection using chest CT scan images (Ali et al. 2020). In recent years, the revolution in neural networks, primarily Deep Learning (DL), has attracted several researchers in developing an intelligent clinical diagnosis system using medical images. Deep-learning architecture has several hidden layers, and each layer can extract information from input data to model the behaviour of the data. Graphical Processing Units (GPU) are used to implement the DL models to discover intricate patterns in the data, since the model needs to process a massive amount of data and demands more computational power for processing data in multiple levels (layers). Therefore, DNNs can extract features that generalize well for unseen scenarios and samples. Besides, DNNs offer a better temporal and spatial resolution to analyze signals compared to conventional machine-learning methods (lin et al. 2020).

The performance of machine-learning and deep-learning algorithms pre-dominantly depends on network hyper-parameters. Because tuning of these network parameters helps the network better to understand the characteristics or patterns of input samples, some of the most common hyper-parameters used in DL models for possible tuning are: (i) a total number of hidden layers; (ii) a maximum number of fully connected layers; (iii) type of activation function in the output layer; (iv) number of training epochs; (v) type of optimization function; (vi) a maximum number of convolutional layers; (vii) batch size; (viii) dropout rate; and (ix) learning rate. These hyper-parameters learn in an iterative fashion using stochastic gradient descent and its variations. Deep-learning techniques, on the other hand, utilize multi-stage hierarchical techniques in which the features are learned directly from the raw signal values, then combined with those extracted from other layers and directly fed to the classifier. Therefore, in addition to providing an algorithm which can be trained directly from the chest CT scan images to labels (COVID-19 or normal or other pneumonia), the features learned in the intermediate stages are designed specifically for the target task.

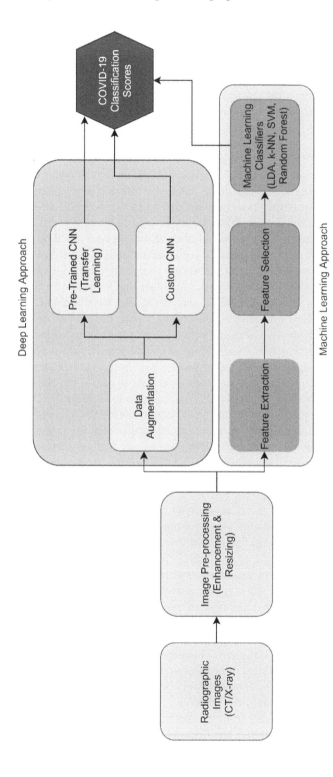

FIGURE.1.3 AI-based COVID-19 disease diagnosis from radiographic-input images of test subjects.

1.4 DATASETS

Image data acquisition is an essential step to design and develop AI-based methods for COVID-19 detection. Lung infection or pneumonia is the most common complication of COVID-19. Chest X-ray and CT are widely-accepted imaging modalities for the diagnosis of lung diseases. Large public CT or X-ray datasets are available for lung diseases. However, the number of CT or X-ray datasets available for the development of AI methods for COVID-19 applications is minimal. Most of the published works so far have used medical images from different websites, and some of the works have used their self-collected images. Table 1.2 reports available datasets from different websites (normal, COVID-19 and other pneumonia) in terms of modality used, number of subjects available. its sources and existing deep-learning models available on websites.

Several deep-learning architectures are deployed for the detection of COVID-19; some of those developed by researchers are listed in Table 1.2. Images used in many of the research works published in the literature were taken from the following two websites

  i. https://github.com/ieee8023/covid-chestxray-dataset (Chest X-ray images)
  ii. https://github.com/UCSD-AI4H/COVID-CT (Chest CT images)

1.5 RELATED RESEARCH

In recent days, researchers started focusing on developing clinical diagnostic tools for early detection of COVID-19 using pathogenic testing, clinical imaging methods, and artificial intelligence to combat the virus. The symptoms and causes of COVID-19 are highly similar to SARS and MERS. In a recent study (Melina et al. 2020), researchers investigated three different types of viruses (SARS, MERS, and COVID-19), their clinical symptoms, and their characteristics. Early detection of COVID-19 and quarantining of the suspects are the most critical actions against COVID-19 to stop spreading the virus and save millions of lives. To date, there is no vaccine or medication invented by scientists or researchers in the world. Due to the limitations of pathogenic testing, clinicians may prefer to detect COVID-19 through clinical imaging methods as the first-line tool for diagnosis (Ho et al. 2020). Among clinical imaging methods, medical images are providing more meaningful information about virus infection and are used more frequently for analyzing disease progression, compared to other imaging methods. Specifically, the performance of chest X-Rays and CT images-based COVID-19 detection system achieved higher sensitivity than RT-PCR tests (Ho et al. 2020). Thereby, medical images are considered promising, accurate, fast, and economical methods of screening and testing COVID-19.

1.5.1 CT Scan Images based COVID-19 Detection using AI Methods

Modified Inception Transfer Learning (MITL) was used to classify COVID-19 or other viral pneumonia using Region of Interest (ROI) features in (Shuai et al. 2020).

TABLE 1.2

Datasets and deep-learning models available

S.No	Modality	Number of Subjects/Images	Reference
1	Chest X-ray	• 219- COVID-19 positive images • 1341 normal images • 1345 viral pneumonia images	https://www.kaggle.com/ tawsifurrahman/covid19- radiography-database
2	Chest X-ray	• 115 – COVID-19 positive images	https://www.sirm.org/category/senza-categoria/covid-19/
3	Chest X-ray	• 542-COVID-19 images from 262 people from 26 countries	https://github.com/ieee8023/covid-chestxray-dataset
4	Chest X-ray	• 8066 normal images • 5538 non-COVID19 pneumonia images • 358 COVID19 images from 266 COVID-19 patient	https://github.com/lindawangg/ covid-net
5	Chest X-ray	CZI 1236 recordsPMC 27337bioRxiv 566medRxiv 361	https://www.kaggle.com/allen-institute-for-ai/CORD-19-research-challenge? select=metadata.readme
6	Chest X-ray	**Testing:** • 234 normal images • 390 pneumonia images **Training:** • 1341 normal images • 3875 pneumonia images **Validation:** • 8 normal images • 8 pneumonia images	https://www.kaggle.com/ paultimothymooney/chest-xray-pneumonia?
7	Chest X-ray	• 7470 – normal chest X-ray images	https://medpix.nlm.nih.gov/home
8	Chest CT	• 349 COVID-19 from 216 patients • 397 non-COVID19 images	https://github.com/UCSD-AI4H/ COVID-CT
9	Chest CT	• 50 lung CT images	http://www.via.cornell.edu/databases/ lungdb.html

Deep-learning models

S.No	Modality	Name of the deep-learning models	Reference
1	Chest X-ray	COVID-RENet, PyTorch based implementation (Custom VGG model)	https://github.com/m-mohsin-zafar/
2	Chest X-ray	DeTrac- Deep CNN approach, called Decompose, Transfer, and Compose.	https://github.com/asmaa4may/DeTrac_covid19
3	Chest CT	ConvNet-PyTorch based implementation	https://github.com/bkong999/covnet
4	Chest X-ray	DarkCOVIDNet- Binary Class and Three class implementation	https://github.com/muhammedtalo/ covid-19

Morphological features such as multiple ground-glass opacities, pseudo cavity, and enlarged lymph nodes from CT scan images are extracted using preprocessing and used as input for training the deep neural network. Maximum classification rates of 89.5% and 79.3%, sensitivity of 88%, and 83%, and specificity of 87%, and 67% are achieved on validation and external dataset, respectively. They used 1065 CT scan images from 219 subjects (COVID-19: 79, and other pneumonia: 180) for developing the deep-learning model for COVID-19 classification.

CT scan images are handy to identify the progression of GGO and mGGO in COVID-19 suspects over a time. Thereby, it provides a way of identifying different stages of COVID-19. The different stages of COVID-19 infections are classified based on the level of severity in the CT scan images. The amount of severity is calculated based on the number of multiple ground-glass opacities in both lungs. These chest CT severity scores are beneficial for clinicians to discover the different stages of COVID-19, such as mild, moderate, severethan classifying COVID-19 or normal (Ran et al. 2020). The researchers used the transfer-learning property a in Convolutional Neural Network (CNN) to classify the input sample into two classes: COVID-19 positive and other viral pneumonia. They achieved a maximum accuracy of 89.5%. The same algorithm gives 79.3% accuracy while testing with the external dataset.

However, researchers have classified the stages of COVID-19 into four: mild; moderate; severe; and critical using serial chest CT scan images and deep-learning models to achieve a maximum mean classification rate of 84.81% in (Lu et al. 2020). A Convolutional Neural Network (CNN) with U-Net architecture is used to differentiate among the four different stages of COVID-19 based on a percentage of opacification score from the segmented chest CT scan images. The two lung regions and five lobes of lung regions are extracted from 126 subjects' CT scans and a group of radiologists. A Likert scale is used to derive the percentage of opacification and group the subjects according to stage.

In another study, researchers utilized ultrasound to observe imaging manifestations of COVID-19 (Yi et al. 2020). They investigated ultrasound images of 20 patients who suffered from mild symptoms; results confirmed that ultrasound sound images captured from posterior and inferior areas of the lung indicate viral infection compared to normal lung images. However, this method may not be useful for diagnosing COVID-19 patients with moderate, severe, or critical symptoms (Lung ultrasound, 2020).

RADLogics brand has developed an intelligent Artificial Intelligence Powered System for detecting COVID-19 using CT scan images; this achieved a maximum sensitivity of 98.2% and specificity of 92.2% when testing the system with 157 patients. This AI system is currently deployed in hospitals in China, Italy, and Russia for combating COVID-19 (Ophir et al. 2020). In Lin et al. (2020), researchers developed a deep-learning network called COVNet as a screening tool for COVID-19 detection. The network utilized visual features from chest CT scan images of COVID-19 pneumonia and non-pneumonia to develop a robust model. The model achieved a maximum sensitivity of 87% and 90% for COVID-19 and other pneumonia detection, respectively. Using AI to develop a frontline tool to assist specialists in diagnosing COVID-19 could save millions of lives. However, developing an intelligent AI-based system requires high-quality clinical data for accurate detection. To develop an intelligent system, the diagnosis system should be trained with a large number of input samples of different types to effectively model the system for better prediction or detection (McCall 2020). Alibaba Research Academy has developed its automated clinical diagnosis system for COVID-19 using artificial intelligence methods, achieved a maximum accuracy of 96% and diagnosed more than 30,000 cases in 26 hospitals in China (Ali et al. 2020).

Wang et al. have developed a fully functional deep-learning model for COVID-19 detection using a large number of chest CT scan images collected from six regional cities in the Republic of China (Wang et al. 2020). A total of 5,372 subjects' chest CT scan images (COVID-19: 1,266 subjects, CT-EGFR (epidermal growth factor receptor): 4106 subjects). Two deep-learning networks, namely, DenseNet-121 and COVID-19Net, are used for extracting the lung area from CT scan, and COVID diagnostics, respectively. Here, two transfer-learning algorithms are used to extract 64-dimensional deep-learning features from DenseNET and combined with clinical features (sex, age, and comorbidity) to develop a multivariate Cox Proportional Hazard (CPH) model to predict chances of the patient needing a long hospital stay to recover. The performances of deep-neural networks are assessed through the Area Under Curve (AUC), and the maximum value of AUC achieved for training, and testing is 0.90, and 0.86, respectively. Besides, the researchers used deep-learning visualization algorithms to identify the most common lung region affected by COVID-19 patients.

The first work on COVID-19 detection by using CNN and conventional machine-learning methods such as Artificial Neural Network (ANN) and Adaptive Neuro-Fuzzy Inference System (ANFIS) is reported in (Singh et al. 2020). The researchers used multiple objective differential evaluation (MODE) to tune the hyperparameters of CNN (batch size, kernel function, epoch, activation function, hidden neurons and convolution filter size and number). The proposed system can classify the severity of the COVID-19 suspects into four different levels: mild; moderate; severe; and critical) and achieved a higher mean classification rate of 93.5% in MODE-CNN compared to conventional CNN (93%), ANFIS (92.1%), and ANN (90.2%).

In Abdullah et al. (2020) the researchers used four image filtering methods such as MPEG7 Histogram filter, Gabor filter, Pyramid of Rotation-Invariant Local Binary Pattern Histograms Image Filter, Fuzzy 64-bin Histogram Image Filter to choose the most selective regions from chest CT scan images of COVID-19 and Severe Acute Respiratory Symptoms (SARS). The proposed work utilizes a limited number of samples (COVID-19: 51 images; SARS: 51 images) to differentiate between COVID-19 or SARS using conventional machine-learning and deep-learning methods. These features are fed into Genetic Algorithm (GA) to find an optimized feature and classified as COVID-19 or SARS using four classifiers: Support Vector Machine (SVM); Naïve Bayes (NB); CNN; and Random Forest (RF)). Maximum mean accuracy of 96.11% is achieved using the RF classifier compared to CNN (94.11%), SVM (86.27%), and NB (86.35%).

Li et al. have used a large number of CT scan images of COVID-19 (n = 1296), Community-Acquired Pneumonia (n = 1735) and non-pneumonia (n = 1325) from

3,322 subjects (male: 1,838, female: 1,484) from six different cities in China to develop an intelligent COVID-19 detection system using a deep-neural network (Li et al. 2020). The U-Net segmentation method is used to preprocess and extract the lung region from the CT scan and to train the CNN. The proposed model achieved a maximum sensitivity of 90% and sensitivity of 96% in detecting COVID-19 and 87% and 90% as sensitivity and specificity of Community Acquired Pneumonia (CAP). Though the system has been trained with larger data, still it does not utilize clinical features to improve robustness.

In Xu (2020), using a 3D-CNN deep neural network, researchers put chest CT scan images into three classes: COVID-19; Influenza-A-viral pneumonia; and healthy. The 3D-CNN model was used to extract multiple cubes from two lung regions based on a location-attention mechanism. Finally, the Bayesian function is used to compute overall infection probability of the chest CT-scan image. The V-Net backbone Inception ResNet (VNET-IR-RPN) model is used to segment the centre image from the input image; data expansion mechanisms (clipping, up-down flipping, and mirroring) are used to increase the larger number of samples of equal size for classification over three types. Finally, classification is performed by using two types of CNN models based on traditional ResNet network architecture, such as ResNet50 and ResNet with Location Attention Mechanism. Finally, the ResNet with location attention mechanism model outperformed the ResNet architecture, giving a maximum mean accuracy of 86.7% for three classes.

In Chen et al. (2020), researchers developed an AI-based COVID-19 diagnosis tool using cloud-based open-access platforms, chest CT scan images and a deep-learning network. The model was developed in such a way that the input CT image is analyzed to find the activation map related to COVID-19 symptoms. It predicted the region in lungs, filtered out unnecessary fields from chest CT scan images, divided the image into four quadrants and analyzed the three consecutive CT images to find lesions. The model was developed and analyzed with retrospective and prospective COVID-19 subjects along with clinical features. The UNet++ model was used for segmenting the infected region in the lungs by searching for ground-glass opacities, and diminutive nodules.

An Artificial Intelligence-inspired Model for COVID-19 Diagnosis and Prediction for Patient Response to Treatment (AIMDP) is proposed in (Elghamrawy et al. 2020). The model has two essential modules; firstly, the diagnosis module, which utilizes a CNN network to process chest CT scan images and diagnose COVID-19. Here, the whale optimization algorithm is used to select the most prominent features of chest CT scan images (such as ground-glass opacity and crazy paving patterns) then feed them into the CNN for COVID-19 detection. The second is the prediction module; in this module, clinical features (sex, age, infection stage, respiratory failure, multi-organ failure and treatment regimens) predict patient response to the given treatment. The conventional ML algorithms such as Support Vector Machine (SVM), Naïve Bayes (NB) classifier, and Discriminant Analysis (DA) methods are used for COVID-19 classification. Noise is filtered from non-lung regions in CT scans and converted into grey-scale images, followed by normalization for reducing the computational complexity of the proposed diagnosis model. Finally, the SVM classifier outperforms NB and

DA classifiers by giving a maximum mean classification rate of 97.14%, compared to 95.99% and 94.71%, respectively.

Researchers used 3-D CNN that combines V-Net architecture with a bottle-neck structure to enhance the quality of chest CT scan images for COVID-19 detection (Shan et al. 2020). Because the raw chest CT scan images usually have low contrast, it is challenging to locate the GGO or mGGO in the scan images. Besides, they used the human-in-the-loop strategy (HITL) to reduce the requirement of a radiologist in locating the infected regions in the lung CT scan images to train the proposed model. They divided the training images into a set of batches; the first batch gets feedback from the radiologist on locating the infected regions in the lung. After that, these images are used to train the model, which will automatically locate the in- fected regions in the second batch. Here, the radiologist corrects any mis- interpretations of the model. It is the first work in COVID-19 detection which utilizes HITL model to develop an intelligent system using chest CT scan images. Two performance measures such as dice- similarity coefficient (DSC), and Pearson correlation coefficient (PCC) are used to classify the COVID-19 subjects into three classes: mild; moderate; and severe. Here DSC is used to measure the percentage of different opinions in detecting infection regions identified by the radiologists and the automated method of detection using a deep-learning model. The POC is used to identify the percentage of lung region infected due to COVID-19, compared to normal lung region. The average value of DSC and POI over three cases are 91.6% and 86.7%, respectively.

He et al. developed an intelligent COVID-19 detection tool using Self-Trans network and chest CT scan images (He et al. 2020). 397 chest CT scans of normal subjects and 349 of COVID-19 patients are used to train, validate and test the system using a transfer-learning approach in different deep-learning architectures, such as VGG16, ResNet18, ResNet50, DenseNet-121, DenseNEt-169, EfficientNet-b0, and EfficientNet-b1. The maximum mean accuracy, Area Under Curve (AUC) and Fl score, of 86%, 0.94 and 0.85, respectively, are achieved using a Self-Trans network with DenseNet-169.

In Amyar et al. (2020), researchers employed Multi-Task Learning (MTL) in a deep-learning network for smaller size chest CT scan images to detect COVID-19. They performed the three tasks in MTL such as classification (COVID19 vs Non-COVID19), lesion segmentation using U-Net, and Image reconstruction. They utilized three international standard databases in their work. The system used for COVID-19 detection involves preprocessing (resize and intensity normalization), segmentation (lesion detection), and classification using a deep-learning network with MTL method. The proposed MTL work with an input image size of 256×256 achieved a maximum mean accuracy of 86%, sensitivity of 94%, specificity of 79% and area under the curve (AUC) of 0.93.

1.5.2   X-Ray Images based COVID-19 Detection using AI Methods

X-ray based COVID-19 detection systems are more popular compared to CT scan images due to cheaper cost, lower radiation, easier operation and less harm (www.siim.org). A group of researchers investigated three different types of deep-neural networks: ResNet50; ResNetV2; and InceptionV3 to detect COVID-19 using chest X-Ray images of 50 subjects (Feng et al. 2020). A maximum mean classification rate of 98%, 97%, and 87% is achieved in classifying normal or COVID-19 using ResNet50, ResNetV2, and Inception V3 networks. In the above work, due to the limitation of input samples, researchers used transfer- learning approaches to train the system with a fewer number of samples, which demands less computational power compared to conventional deep-neural networks. Later, information gained in the pre-trained model on a large dataset is transferred to the model to be trained.

The Darknet-19-based deep-neural network model is considered as two-class (COVID-19 vs no findings) and three class (COVID-19 vs no findings vs pneumonia) classifier using the You Only Look Once (YOLO) real-time object-detection method for COVID-19 detection, which uses chest x-ray images (Ozturk et al. 2020). A maximum mean classification rate of 98.08% for binary classification (COVID-19 vs no findings) and 87.02% for three-class classification (COVID-19 vs no findings vs pneumonia) can achieved. Besides, the heat map method based on Gradient-Weighted Class Activation Mapping (Grad-CAM) is used for transforming the deep-learning model output into images for better diagnosis by radiologists. The proposed model used a limited number of chest x-ray images (1125 chest x-ray images) for developing an intelligent system for COVID-19 detection. The model performs well in binary classification but gives a poor performance in multiple classification by analyzing the COVID-19 images as pneumonia images.

However, in Abbas et al. (2020), researchers proposed the Decompose Transfer Compose (DecTrac) CNN model for classification of COVID-19 and achieved a maximum mean accuracy of 95.12%, with sensitivity and specificity of 97.91% and 91.87%, respectively. In this work, they used three databases for three classes: normal; COVID-19 and Severe Acute Respiratory Syndrome (SARS); and AlexNet to extract the local features. In consequence, they used the Principal Component Analysis (PCA) as a feature-reduction technique to reduce memory requirements of the proposed model and to speed up the computation process. Finally, transfer learning based on the ResNet model is adopted in classification.

In Khan et al. (2020), 150 normal chest x-ray images and 150 COVID-19 chest x-ray images are used to develop a deep-neural network to detect COVID-19 using the Support Vector Machine classifier. Eight different types of deep-neural networks – AlexNet, Google Net, VGG16, VGG19, DenseNet201, ResNet18, ResNet50, InceptioV3 – are used to extract the edge and region-based features of ground-glass opacities and lesions from chest x-ray images. These features are used to form dynamic features by using COVID-RENet and Custom VGGNet and classified into either COVID-19 positive or COVID-19 negative using the Support Vector Machine (SVM) classifier. The maximum mean accuracy, sensitivity and specificity of 98.3%, 100% and 96.67% achieved using the proposed model compared to state-of-the-art works in the literature.

In the case of Sethy et al. (2020), researchers used 11 feature extraction methods with a deep-neural network to extract in-depth features from COVID-19 positive and COVID-19 negative and classified them using an SVM classifier. The eleven feature-extraction methods are: ResNet50; ResNet101; Inception V3; ResNet18;

AlexNet; VGG16; VGG19; Google Net; Xception Net; InceptionresnetV2; and DenseNet201 AlexNet. Finally, ResNet50 and SVM classifier give the maximum mean accuracy, sensitivity, specificity of 95.38%, 95.52% and 91.41%, respectively, compared to other deep features.

The Shallow-CNN model is used to detect COVID-19 using chest x-ray images in Mukherjee et al. (2020). In this work, the x-ray images of different sizes - 100 by 100, 50 by 50, and 150 by 150 - are used to classify patients into either COVID-19 positive or COVID-19 negative using the Shallow-CNN model; the performance of the proposed system is compared with VGG16 and MobileNet. Here, 130 chest images are COVID-19 positive, and 130 are negative (MERS, SARS and ARDS: 51 images; Pneumonia: 48 images; and Normal: 31 images) for developing the proposed model. The maximum mean accuracy of 96.15%, 95%, 50% is achieved for 100 by 100, 50 by 50, and 150 by 150 size chest x-ray images, respectively, using the proposed CNN model. It is important to note that the planned model requires fewer parameters compared to conventional CNN, requires lesser computational memory and computation time and gives higher classification rates.

The Bayesian Optimization Method, based on SqueezeNet, was used for COVID-19 detection in (Ucar et al. 2020). Two different databases are used to collect the x-ray images of COVID-19, normal, and pneumonia for training the model. Augmentation was performed to balance the number of x-ray images for three classes to achieve optimal performance. As a result of augmentation, each class consisted of 1,536 chest x-ray images for training the model, which achieved a maximum mean classification rate, sensitivity and specificity of 98.26%, 98.26% and 99.13%, respectively, compared to other state-of-the-art methods in the literature. Here, normal x-rays consisted of MERS, SARS and ARDS images. The Bayesian optimization method was used to fine-tune the hyperparameters of SqueezeNet to achieve higher accuracy in less computation time. The proposed model achieved 100% accuracy in detecting COVID-19, 98.04% in detecting normal and 96.73% in detecting pneumonia.

The first work on utilizing several machine-learning classifiers and deep-learning network in COVID-19 detection using chest x-ray images is reported in (Kumar et al. 2020). The researchers used two different databases to classify input x-ray images into normal, COVID-19, and pneumonia, using seven classifiers to achieved a good classification accuracy: random forest (97.3%); XGBoost predictive classifier (97.7%); Logistic regression (96.6%); Decision Tree (93.1%); Naïve Bayes (89%); Adaboost (92.1%); and Nearest Neighbor (94.7%). The ResNet152 deep learning architecture was used for training the images, and the imbalanced images in three classes were balanced using Synthetic Minority Oversampling Technique (SMOTE) and classified using machine-learning classifiers.

The Capsule Network's first use in detecting COVID-19 using chest x-ray images is reported in (Afshar et al. 2020). Capsule networks are most useful if the network uses smaller a dataset and a smaller number of tunable parameters, and requires less time for developing decision-making systems. The proposed model classifies the input images into either COVID-19 positive or COVID-19 negative. Here, three different types of chest x-ray images - bacterial, pneumonia and normal- are considered COVID-19 negative. The system was tested with two different conditions - capsule network with pre-trained dataset and capsule network without pre-training – and achieved a maximum mean classification rate of 98.3% and 95.7%, respectively. Though the proposed model gives a higher classification rate with a pre-trained network, the sensitivity of the system is too low compared to the other case (80%).

In Farooq et al. (2020), researchers classified the input chest x-ray images into four classes: normal; bacterial pneumonia; viral pneumonia; and COVID-19 using Residual Network with 50 layers. The images of four classes were acquired from two different databases, and the augmentation process was performed to balance the dataset used for training the proposed model. The network was pre-trained with ImageNet and adopted transfer learning in classifying the images into four classes. The proposed model achieved a maximum mean classification rate of 96.23% and 83.5% on COVID-ResNet50 and COVID-Net, respectively.

Domain Extension Transfer Learning (DETL) was first introduced in Basu et al. (2020) in place of the transfer-learning approach in CNN for COVID-19 detection. In Transfer learning, if the source and target images are different, specifically in medical imaging, the network may learn with the features of two different images. This limitation in transfer learning can be rectified by using domain extension transfer learning on CNN. Three different chest x-ray databases were used to classify the images into four classes: normal; other diseases; pneumonia; and COVID-19. This achieved a maximum mean classification accuracy of 95.3%. Besides, a Gradient Class Activation Mapping (Grad-CAM)-based heat map was used to identify different infection regions from chest x-ray images of COVID-19 compared to other classes. The proposed model utilized ImageNet as the pre-trained network to detect COVID-19. In conclusion, the COVID-19 images indicate that ground-class opacity is the most common clinical indicator which exists in all COVID-19 samples.

Comparing four different pre-trained models on x-ray images classification - ResNet118, SqeezeNet, DenseNet201 and AlexNet - was first used for COVID-19 detection using CNN in Chowdhury et al. (2020). The data-augmentation method was used to achieve a balanced dataset for both training and testing on CNN. Three datasets of chest x-ray images - normal, viral pneumonia and COVID-19 - were used to classify the images into two classes (COVID-19 and normal) and three classes (COVID-19, normal and viral pneumonia); this achieved a maximum mean classification rate of 98.3% and 98.3%, respectively, using the SqueezeNet pre-trained network.

Recently, researchers developed a mobile application to detect COVID-19 based on a snapshot of chest x-ray images called MobileExpert (Li et al. 2020). Here, they used the Knowledge-Transfer Distillation (KTM) method as a medical-screening application and a medical student (MS) network as a mobile-screening application to develop a mobile expert system for COVID-19 detection.

In Narin et al. (2020), three different types of pre-trained deep-neural networks – ResNet50, InceptionV3, and Inceptio-ResNetV2 – were used for COVID-19 detection using chest x-ray images. This work utilized a limited number of chest x-ray samples for detecting COVID-19 (50 x-ray images) or normal (50 x-ray images). Because of the limited number of training samples, the transfer-learning approach was used on three networks, and their performance was compared. Among the three different pre-trained models, ResNet50 outperformed and achieved a higher classification rate of 98% with a specificity of 100%, compared to Inception V3 (97%) and Inception-ResNetV2 (87%).

The first work on Multi-level thresholding with an Otsu-objective function and Support Vector Machine (SVM) based segmentation was performed with chest x-ray images to identify the distinct areas, as reported in Mahdy et al. (2020). Though the proposed model utilized a very limited number of samples (15 normal chest x-ray images and 25 COVID-19 chest x-ray images) from the international standard database, the system achieved a maximum mean classification rate of 95.3% with a sensitivity and specificity of 99.7% and 97.48%, respectively, in classifying normal or COVID-19.

In Wang et al. (2020), researchers developed the first open-source database (COVIDx) for COVID-19 research using a large set of chest x-ray images for pneumonia, normal, and COVID-19 from five data repositories. Though the number of COVID-19 subjects is fewer than normal or pneumonia subjects, this is one of the largest open-source database available for researchers over the world. Besides, the researchers developed a deep-neural network called COVID-Net using a convolutional-neural-network principle. The machine-driven data-exploration strategy for the design of optimal micro and macro architecture of COVID-Net is based on residual projection-expansion-projection-extension (PEPX) design pattern. The performance of the proposed COVID-Net was compared with ResNet50 and VGG-19 architecture and achieved maximum mean classification rates of 93%, 90.6% and 83%, respectively. Besides, the proposed network achieved high sensitivity in detecting pneumonia and COVID-19 compared to the ResNet50 and VGG-19 models.

The first work on detecting the COVID-19 using chest CT scans and chest X-ray images was reported in Maghdid et al. (2020). The proposed model utilized a limited number of samples of normal and COVID-19 from five different databases to develop a COVID-19 detection model. The researchers used the convolutional neural network (CNN) and the modified AlexNet model for COVID-19 detection. Here, transfer-learning methodology is implemented in AlexNet using theImageNet dataset. The Modified AlexNet achieved maximum mean classification rates of 98% and 82% using x-ray images and CT scans, respectively, compared to the CNN (accuracy: 94 (x-ray) and 94.1 (CT scans)).

1.6   CONCLUSION

Recent studies in the literature reported COVID-19 detection using RT-PCR testing and chest X-Ray images with a limited number of subjects. Here, the RT-PCR test is considered as a global standard method of COVID-19 detection, followed by Chest CT-scan and Chest X-ray images. There are a few autonomous COVID-19 detection systems developed based on visual features extracted from chest CT scan images which reported a lower sensitivity and specificity. After the discovery of COVID-19 in late 2019, several research papers were published on COVID-19 detection using multi-modality approaches. Most of the earlier works focussed on regional databases with a limited number of samples, unbalanced datasets, and a limited number of classes (COVID-19 positive or normal). Researchers rarely used AI methods to diagnose COVID-19 using geometric or region of interest (ROI) features from Chest CT-scan and X-ray images. Besides, researchers utilized the original image features to detect COVID-19 compared to the infection-specific or morphological features from CT images, such area, density, size, width, number of GGO, and depth of lesions for diagnosing COVID-19. Recent research works achieved lower sensitivity rate due to the inefficiency of image features in differentiating different types of pneumonia. So, it is crucial to investigate different types of features from chest CT-Scan of COVID-19 pneumonia and other viral pneumonia with normal chest CT scan images of a large group of subjects for developing intelligent and robust clinical diagnosis systems for COVID-19 detection. Earlier works identified COVID-19 based on CT scan images of severe cases only. None of the earlier works focused on identifying COVID-19 based on mild and moderate symptoms. Though numerous works related to deep learning were reported in the literature, most of the work involved a small group of subjects, and the number of images considered for deep learning was limited. Often deep-earning methods based on CNN involves training data of thousands of images of test subjects for reliable performance scores (AI for COVID, 2020). Due to inadequate availability of open datasets for COVID-19, the prediction accuracy of CNN is also limited. Researchers also used data augmentation approaches to increase the size of the training data to improve the prediction scores. However, the models are trained only for a particular cohort of cases, which leads to overfitting of the CNN models (Mei et al. 2020). There is a need to generate a training dataset for COVID-19 which is diverse in the type of test subjects considered based on demographic and geographic information.

ACKNOWLEDGEMENT

This work is financially supported by the Kuwait Foundation for the Advancement of Sciences (KFAS), Kuwait, through an exploratory research grant scheme. Grant Number: CN20-13QE-02.

REFERENCES

Abbas A., Abdelsamea M., Gaber M. M., *Classification of COVID-19 in chest X-ray images using DeTraC deep convolutional neural network, medRxiv*, 1 April 2020, doi: 10.1101/2020.03.30.20047456.

Abdullah F. A., Ibrahim S. G., Awad A. K. H., A novel approach of CT images feature analysis and prediction to screen for corona virus disease (COVID-19). *arXiv*, 2020, doi:10.20944/preprints202003.0284.v1.

Accelerated Emergency Use Authorization (EUA) Summary COVID-19 RT-PCR Test (Laboratory Corporation of America). *Lab Corp COVID-19 RT-PCR test EUA Summary*, 2020.

Afshar P., Heidarian S., Naderkhani F., et al., COVID-CAPS: a capsule network-based framework for identification of COVID-19 cases from X-ray images, arXiv, 2020. (2004.02696v2).

Ali N., Ceren K., Ziynet P., Automatic detection of coronavirus disease (COVID-1919) using X-Ray images and deep convolutional neural networks, arXiv, 2003.10849, Mar 2020.

Amyar A., Modzelewski R., Ruan S., Multi-task deep learning based CT imaging analysis for COVID-19: classification and segmentation, medRxiv, 21 April 2020, doi:10.11 01/2020.04.16.20064709.

Basu S., Mitra S., Saha N., Deep learning for screening COVID-19 using chest X-Ray images, arXiV:2004.10507v3 [eess.IV], 24 April 2020.

Chen J., Wu L., Zhang J., et al., Deep learning-based model for detecting 2019 novel coronavirus pneumonia on high-resolution computed tomography: a prospective study, medRxiv, Mar 2020, doi: 10.1101/2020.02.25.20021568.

Chowdary M. E. H., Rahman T., Khandakar A., et al., Can I help in screening viral and COVID-19 penumonia?, arXiv preprint, 29 Mar 2020.

Chowdhury M. E. H., Rahman T., Khandakar A., MAhar R., et al., Can AI help in screening Viral and COVID-19 pneumonia?, arXiv.2003.12145.v2, 28 April 2020,

Elghamrawy S., Hassanien A. E., Diagnosis and prediction model for COVID-19 patient's response to treatment based on convolutional neural networks and whale optimization algorithm sing CT images, medRxiv, 21 April 2020, doi: 10.1101/2020.04.16.20063990.

Farooq M., Hafeez A., COVID-ResNet: a deep learning framework for screening of COVID19 from radiographs, arXiv:2003.14395v1, 31 Mar 2020.

Feng X., Nannan S., Fei S., et al., Emerging coronavirus 2019-nCoV pneumonia. *Radiology, The Radiology Society of North America*, April 2020. (in press)

Hao W., Li M., Clinical diagnostic value of CT imaging in COVID-19 with multiple negative RT-PCR testing, *Travel Medicine and Infectious Disease*, Mar 2020, doi:10.1016/ j.tmaid.2020.101627.

He X., Yang X., Zhang S., et al., Sample-efficient deep learning for COVID-19 diagnosis based on CT scans. *IEEE Transactions on Medical Imaging*, 17 April 2020, doi:10.11 01/2020.04.13.200063941.

Ho Y. F. W., Hiu Y. S. L., Ambrose H. T. F., Siu T. L., et al., Frequency and distribution of chest radiographic findings in COVID-19 positive patients, radiology. *Radiology Society of North America*, Mar 2020.

Huang, C., Wang, Y., Li, X., et al., Clinical features of patients infected with 2019 novel coronavirus in Wuhan, China. *The Lancet*, 395(10223):497–506, 2020.

Huang Y., Wang S., Liu Y., et al., A preliminary study on the ultrasonic manifestations of peripulmonary lesions of non-critical novel coronavirus pneumonia (COVID-19), 2020. doi.org/10.2139/ssrn.3544750.

Khan S. H., Sohail A., Zafar M. M., Khan A., Coronavirus disease analysis using chest X-ray images and a novel deep convolutional neural network, preprint, April 2020.

Kumar R., Arora R., Bansal V., et al., Accurate prediction of COVID-19 using chest X-Ray images through deep feature learning model with SMOTE and machine learning classifiers, medRxiv, April 17, 2020, doi: 10.1101/2020.04.13.20063461

Li K., Fang Y., Li W., et al. CT image visual quantitative evaluation and clinical classification of coronavirus disease (COVID-19), *European Radiology*, 3: 4407–4416, doi: 10.1007/s00330-020-06817-6.

Li X., Li C., Zhu D., COVID-Mobile expert: on device COVID-19 screening using snapshots of chest X-Ray, arXiv:2004.03042v2, 13 April 2020.

Li F., Dong L., Huadan X., Longjiang Z., Zaiyi L., Bing Z., Lina Z., et al., Progress and prospect on imaging diagnosis of COVID-19-19. *Chinese Journal of Academic Radiology*, 3:4–13, 2020b, doi: 10.1007/s42058-020-00031-5.

Lin L., Lixin Q., Zeguo Z., et al., Artificial intelligence distinguishes COVID-19 from community acquired pneumonia on chest CT. *Radiology, Radiology Society of North America*, Mar 2020. (In press).

Lu H., Rui H., Tao A., Pengxin Y., Han K., Qian T., Liming X., Serial quantitative chest CT assessment of COVID-19: deep-learning approach, Mar 30 2020, doi: 10.1148/ryct.2020200075.

Maghdid H. S., Asaad A. T., Ghafoor K. Z., Sadiq A. S., Khan M. K., Diagnosing COVID-19 pneumonia from X-Ray and CT images using deep learning and transfer learning algorithms, arXiv:2004,00038, Mar 31, 2020.

Mahase, E. Coronavirus: COVID-19 has killed more people than SARS, and MERS combined, despite lower case fatality rate. *The BMJ*, 368:m641, 2020, doi:10.1136/bmj.m641.

Mahdy L. N., Ezzat K. A., Elmousalami H. H., Ella H. A., Hassanien A. E., Automatic X-ray COVID-19 lung image classification system based on multi-level thresholding and support vector machine, medRxiv, April 6, 2020, doi: 10.1101/2020.03.30.20047787.

McCall B., COVID-19 and artificial intelligence: protecting health-care workers and curbing the spread. *Digital Health, The LANCET*, 2: e166–e167, April 2020.

Mei X., Lee H. C., Diao Kyue, Huang M, Lin B, Liu C, et al. Artificial intelligence–enabled rapid diagnosis of patients with COVID-19. *Nature Medicine*, 26:1224–1228, 2020, https://doi.org/10.1038/s41591-020-0931-3.

Melina H., Soheil K., Ali G., Sravanthi R., Lee M., Coronavirus Disease 2019 (COVID-19): lessons from Severe Acute Respiratory Syndrome and middle east respiratory syndrome. *American Journal of Radiology*, 2020. doi: 10.2214/AJR.20.22969.

Mukherjee H., Ghosh S., Dhar A., et al., Shallow convolutional neural network for COVID-19 outbreak screening using chest X-rays, *TechRxiv*, 21 April, 2020, doi: 10.36227/techrxiv.12156522.

Narin A., Kaya C., Pamuk Z., Automatic detection of coronavirus disease (COVID-19) using X-ray images and deep convolutional neural networks, arXiv:2003.10849, 24 Mar 2020.

NIH harnesses AI for COVID-19 diagnosis, treatment, and monitoring | National Institutes of Health (NIH) n.d. https://www.nih.gov/news-events/news-releases/nih-harnesses-ai-covid-19-diagnosis-treatment-monitoring [Retrieved on 30.10.2020].

Ophir G., Maayan F.-A., Hayit G., Patrik D. B., et al., Rapid AI development cycle for the Coronavirus (COVID-19) pandemic: initial results for automated detection and patient monitoring using deep learning CT image analysis, arXIC:2003:05037, 2020.

Ozturk T., Talo M., Azra E., et al., Automated detection of COVID-19 cases using deep neural network with X-Ray images. *Computers in Biology and Medicine*, 121, 2020, doi: 10.1016/j.compbiomed.2020.103792.

Radiology Assistant, https://radiologyassistant.nl/chest/lk-jg-1 [Retrieved on 3 April 2020].

Ran Y., Xiang L., Huan L., Yanling Z., Xianxiang Z., Qiuxia X., Yong L., Cailiang G., Wenbing Z., Chest C. T. Severity score: an imaging tool for assessing severe COVID-19. *Radiology*, 295(1) : 202–207, 2020.

Sana, S., Aidin A., Sudheer B., Ali G., Coronavirus disease 2019 (COVID-19): a systematic review of imaging findings in 919 patients, *American Journal of Roentgenology, AJR*, 215:1–7, 2020.

Sethy P. K., Behera S. K., Detection of coronavirus disease (COVID-19) based on deep features, preprints, 19 Mar 2020, doi: 10.20944/preprints202003.0300.v1.

Shan F., Gao Y., Wang J., Shi W., et al., Lung infection quantification of COVID-19 in CT images with deep learning, 2020.

Shuai W., Bo K., Jinlu M., Xianjun Z., Mingming X., Jia G., Mengjiao C., Jingyi Y., Yaodong L., Xiangfei M., Bo X., A deep learning algorithm using CT images to screen for Corona Virus Disease (COVID-19). *medRxiv*, 2020, doi: 10.1101/2020.02.14 .20023028.

Singh D., Vaishali, V. K., Kaur M., Classification of COVID-19 patients from chest CT images using multi-objective differential evolution–based convolutional neural networks, *European Journal of Clinical Microbiology & Infectious Diseases*, 2020, doi: 10.1007/s10096-020-03901-z.

Soon H. Y., Kyung H. L., Jin Y. K., et al., Chest radiographic and CT findings of the 2019 novel coronavirus disease (COVID-19): analysis of nine patients treated in Korea, Korean. *Journal of Radiology*, 21(4):494–500, 2020.

Stoecklin, S. B., Rolland, P., Silue, Y., et al., First cases of coronavirus disease 2019 (COVID-19) in France: surveillance, investigations and control measures, January 2020. *Eurosurveillance*, 25(6):2000094, 2020.

Ucar F., Korkmaz D., COVIDiagnostics-Net: deep bayes-squeezeNet based diagnostic of the coronavirus disease 2019 (COVID-19) from X-Ray images. *Medical Hypotheses*, 2020, doi: 10.1016/j.mehy.2020.109761.

University of California San Diego CT Scan Image Database, https://github.com/UCSD-A14H/COVID-19-CT.

Wang L., Lin Z. Q., Wong A., COVID-Net: a tailored deep convolutional neural network design for detection of COVID-19 cases from Chest X-Ray images, arXiv:2003.09871v4, 11 May 2020a.

Wang S., Zha Y., Li W., Wu Q., Li X., et al., A fully automatic deep learning system for COVID-19 diagnostic and prognostic analysis, *medrXiv*, https://doi.org/10.1101/202 0.03.24.20042317, 2020c.

Wang, Y., Hu, M., Li, Q., Zhang, X. P., Zhai, G., and Yao, N. Abnormal respiratory patterns classifier may contribute to large-scale screening of people infected with COVID-19 in an accurate and unobtrusive manner. arXiv preprint arXiv: 2002.05534, 1–6, 2020b.

Wei-cai D., Han-wen Z., Juan Y., Hua-jian X., et al., CT imaging and differential diagnosis of COVID-19. *Canadian Association of Radiologists Journal*, 1–6, 2020, doi: 10.1177/ 0846537120913033.

WHO Coronavirus Disease (COVID-19) Dashboard | WHO Coronavirus Disease (COVID-19) Dashboard n.d. https://covid19.who.int/ [Retrieved on 26.10.2020]. www.SIIM.org.

Xu X., Jiang X., Ma C., Du P., et al., Deep learning system to screen coronavirus disease 2019 pneumonia, arXiv:2002.09334, 22 April 2020.

Ying Z., Yang-Li L., Zi-Ping L., Jian-Yi K., Xiang-Min L., You-You Y., Shi-Ting F., Clinical and CT imaging features of 2019 novel coronavirus disease (COVID-19). *Journal of Infection*, 26 February 2020, doi: 10.1016/j.jinf.2020.02.022.

2 Review on Imaging Features for COVID-19

D. Chitradevi[1] and S. Prabha[2]
[1]Department of CSE, Hindustan Institute of Technology and Science, dcdevi@hindustanuniv.ac.in
[2]Department of ECE, Hindustan Institute of Technology and Science, sprabha@hindustanuniv.ac.in

2.1 INTRODUCTION

Coronaviruses were surrounded by positive RNA (Ribonucleic Acid) which range from 60 nm to 140 nm of diameter. There are four types of coronaviruses: HKU1 (HCoV-HKU1); NL63; 229E; and OC43, all of which are circulated in humans. HKU1 is a species of coronaviruses in humans which is a novel representative of group II (beta) from an adult, NL63 is a novel representative of a group I (alpha) from a child with bronchiolitis, 229E and OC43 are representative of group I (alpha) and II (beta) viruses, which are common cold viruses (Pyrc et al., 2007). The Human coronavirus OC43 (HCoV-OC43) causes problems in respiratory systems. Initially, the coronavirus β genera originated from bats and traversed to humans via intermediate hosts of civet cats in China. These viruses are designated as SARS-CoV-2. During 2012, the MERS-CoV has emerged from bats and dromedary camels as intermediate hosts. This has developed into a new public health disease. HCoV-NL63, HCoV-229E and HCoV-OC43 are SARS-CoV-2, and HCoV-HKU1 is MERS-CoV (Singhal, 2020).

For the past two decades, coronavirus has been related to noteworthy disease outbreaks in East Asia and the Middle East (Sheng 2020). In 2012, SARS and MERS emerged. At the end of year 2019, a new coronavirus was named SARS- CoV-2, which occurred in Wuhan, China. This led to an outbreak of rare viral pneumonia. It is extremely transmissible and known as COVID-19. Nowadays, COVID-19 is extremely epidemic and it poses an extraordinary hazard to public health.

Currently, health care workers are giving their full efforts and support to control this epidemic. In February, 2020, the World Health Organization (WHO) published the authorized name for the current coronavirus as COVID-19, which is produced by SARS-CoV-2 (Hageman, 2020; Sun et al., 2020; Kuldeep et al., 2020). Originally, a group of coronavirus patients was identified in the Huanan South China Seafood marketplace in Wuhan (Gralinski and Vineet, 2020). Coronavirus is in the Coronaviridae group and the Coronavirinae subgroup. The novel coronavirus is genetically distinct. Up to 2020, there were six Covs known to infect humans (Fan et al., 2019). COVID-2019 disease emerged in China and spread rapidly to other countries.

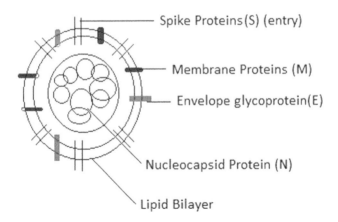

FIGURE 2.1   Structure of the coronavirus.

The severity of the disease and its rapid spread spurred WHO to announce a global health emergency day on 31ˢᵗ January, 2020. Afterwards, a pandemic situation was declared on 11ᵗʰ March, 2020. At present, there is no effective treatment for COVID-19, since there is no approved vaccination or drugs for giving humans with coronavirus infections. Currently all nations are working hard to prevent the further spread of COVID-19 (Kuldeep et al., 2020).

Coronaviruses is encoded with four major structural proteins, namely, S-spike, M-membrane, E-envelope, and N-nucleocapsid. These proteins play a major role in viral replication. SARS-CoV-2 contains 8b protein. S protein is the entry point of the infection, M-protein is a abundant viral protein, E-is the smallest protein and N-is a single-standard positive RNA genome, as represented in Figure 2.1 (Kuldeep et al., 2020).

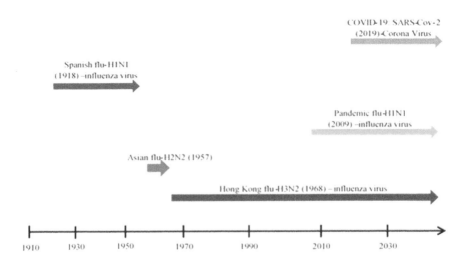

FIGURE 2.2   Five pandemics since 1918 and globally-circulated viruses.

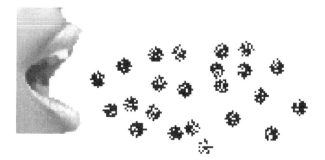

FIGURE 2.3   Transmission of coronavirus through airborne droplet.

COVID-19 has been categorized as a pandemic along with those shown in Figure 2.2: 1918 was called Spanish flu; H1N1, Asian flu; H2N2-1957, in 1968, Hong Kong flu; and H3N2, Pandemic flu; and H1N1, in 2009, which caused approximately 50, 1.5, 1, and 80% of human deaths, respectively (Simonsen et al., 1998; Johnson and Mueller, 2002; Kain and Fowler, 2019).

The major indications of COVID-19 viruses are sore throat, cough, breathlessness, fever,and fatigue among others. These are mild in most people, though in older people it may develop into acute respiratory, multi-organ dysfunction, pneumonia, and distress syndrome (ARDS). Many people are asymptomatic (Cheng and Shan 2020). People of all ages are vulnerable. Infection can be transferred via large droplets produced through coughing and sneezing by symptomatic patients; however, it can also come from those who are asymptomatic (World Health Organization Situation Reports, 2020). Based on the review report, viral loads are identified from symptomatic and asymptomatic people by comparing nasal cavity and throat, as displayed in Figure 2.3.

Infected patients have symptoms until they recover. Some people are super spreaders; they spread infected droplets (Figure 2.3) in the air. The infected droplets may live 2 m in the air which spreads over surfaces. In this situation, the virus will continue to live on surfaces for days in favourable atmospheric conditions, though it can be demolished within a minute using common disinfectants like sodium hypochlorite, hydrogen peroxide, etc. Contagion happens when these surfaces are touched before touching the mouth, eyes or nose, or droplets are inhaled. The coronavirus can spread through airborne zoonotic droplets. The coronavirus replicated in the ciliated epithelium, resulting in cellular damage and infection at the infection site. Based on a report published in 2019, Angiotensin is converted into enzyme 2 (ACE.2), which is the coronavirus entry point in human cells (De Souza et al., 2007; Letko et al., 2020). Ways of coronavirus transmission are represented in the Figure 2.3 and Figure 2.4.

Presently, trans-placental transmission from mother to fetus is not defined, but neonatal disease to post-natal transmission has been defined (Chen et al., 2020). Due to this transmission, incubation times differ from 2 to 14 days (median 5 days). Studies have also shown that the ACE2-angiotensin receptor 2 and the virus arrive in the respirational mucosa (Cheng and Shan, 2019).

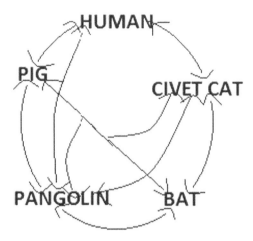

FIGURE 2.4   Major targets of the coronavirus.

Imaging features of ARDS (Das et al., 2017), chronic phases of MERS and SARS are complex which is generic (Das et al., 2016; Ketai et al., 2006). Initially, the imaging findings of COVID-19 were announced with nonspecific results (Chan et al., 2020; Chung et al., 2020). An effort was made to investigate imaging features and characters of the coronavirus syndrome. Radiologists have prepared COVID-19 incidence reports as they help to identify the clinical features and etiology (reason behind this disease). TThe emerging COVID-19 outbreak can be managed with the assistance of pulmonary syndromes.

2.2 REVIEW OF LITERATURE

Coronavirus has spherical/pleomorphic, covered, single-stranded, and enveloped RNA with club-modelled glycoprotein. It has subtypes. The subtypes of coronaviruses are alpha (α), beta (β), gamma (γ) and delta (δ). Each subtype has numerous serotypes. Humans are affected by some subtypes; others affect pigs, cats, birds, dogs and mice. Initially, this virus was treated as a non-fatal, simple virus in 2002. Afterwards, it started spreading to various countries, namely, America, Singapore, Hong Kong, Taiwan, Thailand and Vietnam. In 2003, more than 1,000 patients were affected by SARS-Cov; it was called the black year of the microbiologist. In 2004, WHO announced a "state of emergency" for disease control and prevention. Several infected patients' deaths were reported by Saudi Arabia in 2012. Afterwards, COVID-19 was identified and emerged from Wuhan city (Kumar, 2020).

Numerous reviews were conducted by different authors. They determined that chest CT was one of the best tools to diagnose COVID-19; it is still currently used. (Singhal, 2020; Gralinski and Vineet, 2020; Falaschi et al., 2020). Liu et al. (2020) discussed the origin, evolution and basic properties of COVID-19. The author concluded that these factors are critical in antiviral designs and vaccine development. Furthermore, a comprehensive review was conducted on the basic biology of SARS-CoV-2 by Chauhan (2020). Every week, WHO updates the coronavirus' death rates situation report from the national authorities (World Health Organization, 2020). According to the Commission on Human Medicine's (CHM) advice (14 April), there is no sufficient proof to make a connection between NSAIDs/ibuprofen and vulnerability to COVID-19. Paracetamol or ibuprofen can be taken by patients for COVID-19 (Chaplin, 2020). Fang et al. (2020) showed imaging features of COVID-19 virus infection and RT-PCR with 51 patients' record; they achieved better identification in CT (Fang et al., 2020). CT displays sensitivity of 90% and specificity of 95% in diagnosing COVID-19 pneumonia, higher than what was found in previous studies, particularly taking epidemiological and clinical features into an account (Falasch et al., 2020). Similarly, CT imaging proved a better method for finding COVID-19 features by various authors (Giannitto et al., 2020; Dos Santos, 2020).

A review was conducted to analyse the SARS and MERS outbreaks,which helps radiologists to understand COVID-19 (Hosseiny et al., 2020). The author discussed the history of COVID-19 and current knowledge on drugs, giving updated and consolidated information (Dos and Gouvea, 2020, Xiong et al., 2020). This information includes clinical history, imaging features and laboratory findings of COVID-19 in pregnant patients. Various modalities are available to diagnose COVID-19; however, Chest CT plays an important role in analysing the coronavirus (Guan et al., 2020b).

2.3 DIAGNOSIS

In the past few decades, new diseases have emerged, namely, Ebola virus, Zika virus, Nipah virus, and Coronaviruses (CoVs), which have occurred in different areas. The recent virus is Coronavirus which was spread from Wuhan, China. The genomic-sequencing data of COVID-19 doesn't match with previous Coronaviruses because it was termed novel COVID. This virus is also called as SARS-CoV-2. It originated from a zoonotic host and was transmitted to humans. COVID-19 has lower pathogenesis and higher transmission rates, which is proven across the globe (Dhama et al., 2020). The next generation will facilitate and identify the pathogen in an early stage using real-time PCR. This chapter addresses clinical features and preventive measures for coronaviruses which were globally recommended (Kuldeep et al., 2020).

The COVID-19 clinical features vary from an asymptomatic state to ARDS and multi-organ dysfunction. The important clinical properties are fatigue, myalgia, headache, cough, breathlessness, sore throat and fever. Generally, COVID-19 patients have fever (85%), cough (70%) and shortness of breath (43%); however, abdominal and other asymptomatic symptoms are often appropriate. Conjunctivitis has also been defined as indistinguishable from other respiratory infections. Finally, the disease may progress to respiratory failure, pneumonia and death. These progressions are associated with a marked increase in inflammatory cytokines (Chen et al., 2020). The intermediate time of symptoms is dyspnea: fifth day, hospitalization: seventh day and eighth day: ARDS. In the disease progression, 25–30% of affected patients require intensive care. Complications includes ARDS, acute lung injury, acute kidney injury and other complications, namely, cardiac, cardiovascular or acute stroke. During the second and third week, patients start recovering; such recovery may be extensive. Unfavourable outcomes and death are more common for elderly people (Coronavirus Outbreak, 2020).

COVID-19 patients may be asymptomatic; sometimes a suspected patient is a confirmed patient who was analysed with a molecular test. Coronavirus is diagnosed by molecular tests on respiratory or stool samples; severe cases are detected from blood. The other diagnosis methods for COVID-19 are platelet count, white cell count, C-reactive protein (CRP) and Erythrocyte Sedimentation Rate (ESR), which are non-specific. If the white cell count is less than 1,000, a severe disease called lymphopenia is present. CRP and ESR are the oldest blood tests used to analyse inflammation in the body. Generally these tests are used for determining elevated high procalcitonin level which leads to bacterial co-infection (Singhal, 2020).

Clinical analysis of COVID-19 is non-specific, but diagnosis can be established by a positive RT-PCR test. According to radiologists and a WHO report, RT-PCR is a highly-specific test for diagnosing COVID-19; however, sensitivity is low due to the failure of nucleic acid extraction (Manna et al., 2020). In the US, computed tomography (CT) and chest radiography (CXR) are not officially accepted to diagnose COVID-19. They are less frequently used to diagnose the severity of the disease and determine treatment 2020). A primary tool in early diagnosis of COVID-19 is chest ultrasonography, which was suggested in the United States (Buonsenso et al., 2020). Positron Emission Tomography (PET) has also been explored for COVID-19 diagnosis; it helps detect inflammation and track the progression of this virus (Zou and Zhu, 2020).

Imaging has been evaluated by using the subsequent attributes. Generally, the lesions are split into the lower right, upper right, lower left, and right middle lobes; these are sub-divided into peribronchovascular, diffuse and subpleural. GGO mentions an area of improved attenuation which obscures the underlying pulmonary vessels (Hansell et al., 2008) and is categorized as round or patchy.

There are various modalities recommended to diagnose the progression of COVID-19: Chest Radiography, Positron Emission Tomography/Computed Tomography (PET/CT), Ultrasonography and CT; these identify changes and side effects of COVID-19.

The PCR test takes samples from a person's throat or nose. Saliva may also be investigated for genetic material of COVID-19. This test is very particular, but its sensitivity is 65-95%. According to the sensitivity report, the results may be negative even if the patient is ill. An additional problem with this test is its waiting time, at least 24 hours. Only if the individual is infected can this test be performed. The accuracy of this test is not very high. Figure 2.5 shows the steps of a PCR test.

2.3.1 RT-PCR Test

The spread of COVID-19 from person to person is primarily through respirational droplets, which have a median incubation period of four days (Li et al., 2020). Currently, RT-PCR is considered the gold standard for COVID-19 identification. RT-PCR examinations typically take only a few hours to complete, though

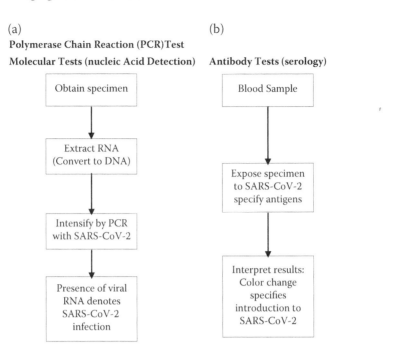

(a)
Polymerase Chain Reaction (PCR)Test
Molecular Tests (nucleic Acid Detection)

(b)
Antibody Tests (serology)

FIGURE 2.5   Steps for processing PCR test (a) Molecular test (b) Antibody test.

additional time is required to transport and prepare the sample. The time required for diagnosis in RT-PCR testing has been extended by an international shortage of personal protective equipment (PPE). The overall positive rate of RT-PCR was reported to be from 30% to 90% at initial stage depending on the respiratory site (Yang et al., 2020). In the current environment of overburdened laboratories, chest computed tomography (Chest CT) is a fast screening test for COVID-19 diagnosis. Furthermore, the RT-PCR test is expensive; it also requires an RNA-mining machine, trained technicians and a laboratory. The chemical costs are high, as are those of the elements required.

2.3.2   CHEST RADIOGRAPHY

The most common imaging test for patients with COVID-19 is portable chest radiography (CXR). Unfortunately, numerous patients test positive (+ve) for COVID-19 with PCR testing , but negative for CXR. This may be due to the lack of lung involvement and data acquisition regarding the disease, or limited access to Personal Protective Equipment. Therefore, the CXR is insensitive for early diagnosis of COVID-19 but, it helps to find baseline information and track disease progression. CXR can diagnose 59% of COVID-19-related abnormalities (Czawlytko et al., 2020; Guan et al., 2020b).

CXR abnormalities with bilateral lower zone peripherally-predominant consolidation and hazy opacities are shown Figure 2.6 (https://github.com/ieee8023/covid-chestxray-dataset, https://aimi.stanford.edu/research/public-datasets). Serial portable

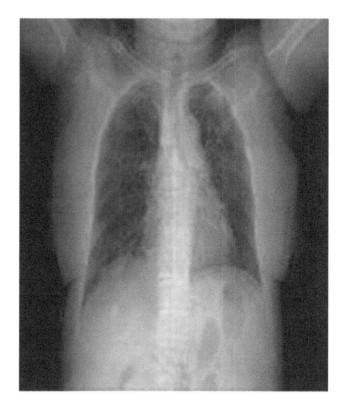

FIGURE 2.6   COVID-19 image from Chest Radiograph.

CXR helps treatment team members and radiologists monitor disease progression within the lungs. In addition, tubes, lines, and complicated processes including sub-cutaneous emphysema, pneumomediastinum, and pneumothorax have been assessed.

2.3.3   PET/CT

PET/CT helps identify the inflammatory processes of the lungs and track disease progression. Sometimes during viral infection, the host response acti-vates inflammatory mediators, such as monocytes, chemokines and neutrophils. Neutorphils depend on the glycolysis, which maintains cellular activity. PET/CT can examine the whole body, which helps to assess the chronic end organ com-plications and incidental results of COVID-19. This is used regularly for in on-cology. It contains previous history reports related to incidental discovery of COVID-19 pneumonia.

2.3.4   MAGNETIC RESONANCE IMAGING (MRI)

Nowadays pulmonary MR imaging features diagnose risks related to COVID-19. MRI has been used to find incidental complicatations in the pulmonary parenchyma, such as cardiac, upper abdominal and vascular. Generally, MRI observes parenchymal changes of COVID-19 pneumonia; it displays as abnormal in both T1 and T2 weighted MR images. These images show consolidative opacities seen in CT and CXR. Cardiac MRI can be used to diagnose cardiomyopathy and myocarditis for COVID-19 patients. The advantage of COVID-19 diagnosis through cardiac MRI is that, it shows global or regional wall motion abnormalities and damage rise in T1 relaxation values. It also signals hyper-intensity demonstrating edema on ECG gated black blood T2 weighted MRI sequences.

2.3.5 ULTRASONOGRAPHY

Chest ultrasonography is helpful in Point of Care (POC) , mainly used to evaluate emergency and intensive care patients (Copetti, 2016). Several reports for imaging acute respiratory failure have been developed, and they have advised the Emergency Department to set up a system to diagnose COVID-19 pneumonia (Peng et al., 2020). Peng et al., 2020 found that ultrasound can be used to monitor recruitment manoeuvres and guide prone positioning.

2.3.6 CHEST COMPUTED TOMOGRAPHY (CT)

CXR is an adequate assessment and screening tool for COVID-19 is CXR, and used for most patients. Chest CT, however, is extremely sensitive and has an accuracy rate of 97% in finding infected patients. According to guidelines from the Centers for Disease Control and Prevention (CDC), viral nuclei acid testing samples are extracted from the respiratory tract. RT-PCR accuracy is 93% for bronchoalveolar lavage fluid sampling, 63% for nasal swab sampling, and 32% for pharyngeal swab sampling (Czawlytko et al., 2020). Like CXR, RT-PCR is more sensitive, though it requires more time (serveral weeks) to test patients. Therefore, most radiologists use CT imaging to identify COVID-19 (Ai et al., 2020). According to a Chinese report, CT has achieved higher sensitivity for analysing COVID-19, compared to RT-PCR examinations; this is strongly accepted by China's National Health Commission. Chest CT results of viral pneumonia are key diagnostic tools for COVID-19 diagnosis. Usual symptoms for COVID-19 are cold, cough, fever and breathing problems. Initially, radiologists suggest chest X-ray, since Ground Glass Opacities (GGO) are a common finding in infected patients. In a GGO pattern, some portions of the lungs are a hazy shade of grey, instead of black with fine white lung markings for blood vessels - a bit like frosted glass (Figure 2.7). However the chest X-ray is not sensitive for COVID-19.

Chest CT shows more detailed information than chest X-ray, as shown in Figure 2.8 (https://github.com/ieee8023/covid-chestxray-dataset/blob/master/). The best CT indicators of COVID-19 are GGO distributed throughout the lungs. Tiny air sacs, or alveoli, get filled with fluid and change to a shade of grey in CT scans (Figure 2.9) (https://www.eurekalert.org/pub_releases/2020-05/mrap-csd050820.php). The imaging structure of COVID-19 in chest-CT contains bilateral, multilobe, rounded GGO, predominantly in the lower lung zone, and having peripheral distribution, with or without consolidation (Zu et al., 2020; Bernheim et al., 2020).

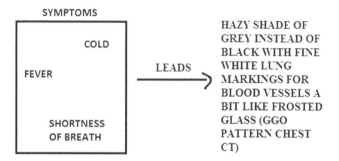

FIGURE 2.7   Representation of Ground Glass Opacities.

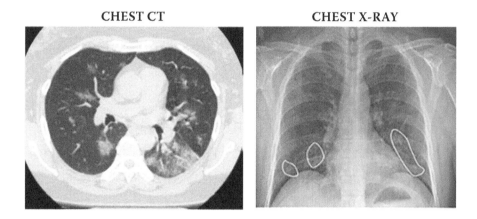

FIGURE 2.8   The detailed view of Chest CT compared to Chest X-ray.

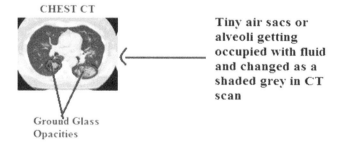

FIGURE 2.9   Tiny air sacs fill with fluid and change to a shade of grey in CT scan.

In severe cases, more and more fluid fills the lobes of the lungs. Finally, the GGO's appearance will be a solid white "consolidation" (Figure 2.10) (https://github.com/ieee8023/covid-chestxray-dataset/blob/master/). Final stages of COVID-19 reveal a crazy-paving pattern. Crazy paving means, there are thickened intralobular and interlobular lines in the GGO pattern. This pattern occurs in a later stage and is identified

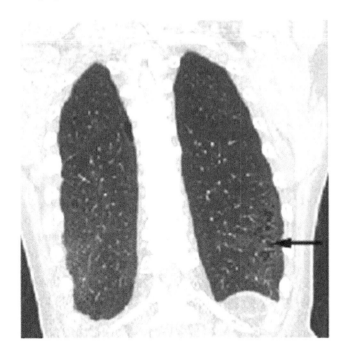

FIGURE 2.10   Severely infected patient representation "Solid White Consolidation".

by inflammation of the interstitial space along with the walls of the lung lobules. This makes the walls heavier and thicker with white lines against the hazy GGO back-ground. It looks like irregularly-shaped stones used to pave a street. Hence it is called crazy paving. Totally, there are three stages of CT findings: GGO; consolidation; and crazy-paving patterns. The combination of all three helps diagnose COVID-19 using imaging (Figure 2.11).

GGO are first signs of COVID-19. Followed by GGO, the other two findings will also be used to diagnose COVID-19. Usually, these findings occur in multiple lobes throughout the lungs, affecting the periphery, or outermost part of the lungs. If patients are in mild or recovering stages of COVID-19, the findings should be isolated into one lobe. Patients who are severely affected will have extreme results on chest CT, which will help to increase the gradual resolution of the ground glass and consolidations.

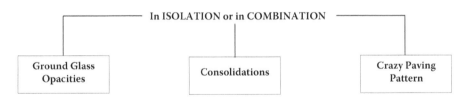

FIGURE 2.11   Chest CT findings of COVID-19.

Due to its involvement in the respiratory system, chest CT has been strongly suggested for suspected COVID-19 patients' initial examination and continuation (Jin et al., 2020). Chest radiographs are used for little diagnostics in the early stages, while CT findings may present right before the onset of symptoms (Kim et al., 2020b). During the intermediate and advanced levels of this disease, CXR shows the progression of ARDS.

Various studies suggest that the better tool for early detection of COVID-19 is chest CT with limited RT-PCR (Corman et al., 2020). Generally, disease progression and severity are critical and demand thorough imaging features. Radiologists should know about patterns and features of COVID-19. Various imaging features have been identified for similar coronavirus-associated syndromes. Because of the COVID-19 outbreak, chest-CT is an essential and effective testing tool. Therefore, this work analyses imaging features for COVID-19 patients.

Generally, there are some key findings, such as pleural effusions, large lymph nodes and lung cavities, which are not seen in COVID-19 (Figure 2.12) (https://www.eurekalert.org/pub_releases/2020-05/mrap-csd050820.php). Pleural effusions are collections of fluid in the pleural space right outside of the lungs. This is common in congestive heart failure and bacterial pneumonia. Large lymph nodes are in the central part of the lungs; they are common in other types of pneumonia. Finally, lung cavities usually develop in fungal and bacterial pneumonia due to necrosis. Even though a chest-CT is very sensitive for COVID-19, the key findings are GGO, considerations and crazy paving. These are also key findings for other diseases, such as pneumonia, influenza and adenovirus. It is also seen in non-infectious conditions, as represented in Figure 2.13 (https://www.eurekalert.org/pub_releases/2020-05/mrap-csd050820.php).

Chest CT abnormalities related to COVID-19 are diagnosed after clinical symptoms. Based on the study that Bernheim et al. (2020) have done about patient symptoms, 44% of patients show symptoms within two days. Through abnormal chest CT, 91% of patient's symptoms have been seen within 3–5 days. After six

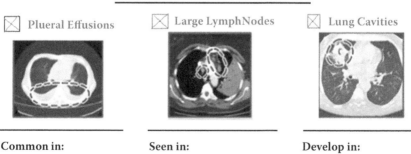

USUALLY NOT SEEN in COVID-19

| ☒ Plueral Effusions | ☒ Large LymphNodes | ☒ Lung Cavities |

Common in:	**Seen in:**	**Develop in:**
• Congestive Heart failure	• Other Pneumonias	• Bacterial &Fungal Pneumonia
• Bacterial Pneumonia		

FIGURE 2.12   The key findings which are not considered for COVID-19.

COVID-19 KEY FINDINGS ALSO SEEN IN...

VIRAL PNEUMONIA
  * Influenza
  * Adenovirus
NON-INFECTIOUS
CONDITIONS

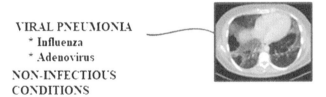

FIGURE 2.13   Key findings which is considered for COVID-19

days, the 96% of symptoms has been shown. Shi et al. identified GGO in 14/15 (93%) asymptomatic healthcare employees with confirmed COVID-19 (Shi et al., 2020). Generally, chest CT is sensitive and non-specific; therefore, patients with these findings should get further clinical evaluation and lab tests to exclude other causes, as displayed in Figure 2.13 (https://www.eurekalert.org/pub_releases/2020-05/mrap-csd050820.php).

Multimodality imaging such as Chest Radiography, Computed Tomography, Positron Emission Tomography/Computed Tomography, Magnetic Resonance Imaging, PCR test and RT-PCR test have been reviewed. Pulmonary features of various imaging modality are described in Table 2.1. Imaging features of CT findings are mentioned in the Table 2.2. A standardised report was created by the Radiology Society of North America (RSNA) advising radiologists to follow a template to improve communication, leading to more efficient patient care (Simpson et al., 2020). SARS-CoV-2 typically has non-specific symptoms, including fever, shortness of breath (respiratory problems), cough and fatigue (Guan et al., 2020b; Huang et al., 2020). Gastrointestinal manifestations, such as diarrhea, nausea and vomiting, are shown in Table 2.3. The findings of COVID-19 overlap with other respirational viral illnesses, highlighting the complexity of diagnostic testing and medical imaging (Czawlytko et al., 2020).

Based on the pros and cons of the above modalities, Radiologic Societies advise caution in screening the imaging features of alleged COVID-19 patients. The American College of Radiology (ACR) has recommended chest CT as a first test to diagnose COVID-19 features. This modality is reserved for symptomatic and hospitalized patients, which is important for clinical analysis. The ACR will suggest compact CXR in ambulatory care assistance when it is medically essential. Patients with mild respiratory features show imaging under the following circumstances. In patients with moderate COVID-19-like respiratory symptoms, imaging should be obtained in the following situations. Regardless of COVID-19 test results, the patient with mild indications needs a clinical report in the next step.

Imaging is obtained from patients with mild, moderate or severe features of COVID-19, irrespective of the outcomes or availability of COVID-19 testing. Imaging permits risk stratification, baseline analysis, identification of an alternative diagnosis and assessment of underlying cardiopulmonary abnormalities in patients who have tested –ve (negative) for COVID-19. In patients who have screened –ve (negative) for COVID-19, imaging allows for risk stratification, baseline

TABLE 2.1

Pulmonary features of different imaging modalities

Modality	Pulmonary findings		
	Acute	Progressive	Recovery
Radiography	1. Peripheral, basilar predominant hazy lung opacities 2. May be unilateral or bilateral	1. Irregular consolidative opacities 2. May become diffuse (ARDS)	Continued vs residual vs resolving opacities
Computed Tomography (CT)	Subpleural ground glass opacity	1. Diffuse ground glass opacity 2. Crazy paving 3. Dense Consolidation 4. Parenchymal bands	1. Progressive absorption 2. Widespread ground glass opacity3)
PET/CT	1. Radiotracer uptake corresponding to ground glass opacities on CT 2. Mediastinal lymphahadenopathy	N/A	N/A
Ultrasound	1. Thickened pleural line 2. Small consolidation 3. Multifocal, confluent, discrete	Alveolar interstitial syndrome	1. Pleural line thickening/uneven 2. B-lines
MRI	1. Increased signal intensity within the affected lung parenchyma	N/A	N/A

examination, alternative diagnosis detection, and evaluation of underlying cardio-pulmonary abnormalities.

2.4   PREVENTION MECHANISMS

COVID-19 virus is a type of human and animal pathogen. It is enclosed with positive-stranded RNA viruses. Coronaviruses are types of betavirus designated by the Study Group of the ICTV as SARS-CoV-2. Another type of betavirus is MERS, which is distantly related (Lu et al., 2020; Zhu et al., 2020). These two viruses have a very close RNA-sequence similarity, which is the key source of COVID-19. It is transmitted directly to bats. The current situation of COVID-19 is that, treatments are not approved due to the progression of viral infections. The prevention of this virus is very difficult due to its non-specific features, infectivity before symptoms, transmission of viruses from asymptomatic persons and

TABLE 2.2

Imaging pattern for CT analysis related to COVID-19 (Czawlytko et al., 2020)

COVID-19 Pneumonia	Justification	CT Results	Recommended Reports
Typical structure/ appearance	Frequently stated imaging aspects of better specificity of COVID-19 pneumonia.	• Bilateral, peripheral, visible intralobular lines ("crazy-paving") / GGO with consolidation. • Multifocal GGO of rounded morphology • Reverse halo sign	Frequently stated imaging aspects of (COVID-19) pneumonia are available. Additional processes are organizing pneumonia and influenza pneumonia, it creates a similar imaging pattern."
Indeterminate structure/ appearance	Non-specific imaging aspects of COVID-19 is pneumonia	• Nonappearance of distinctive aspects AND appearance of diffuse, Multifocal, unilateral or perihilar, lack of specific distribution in GGO (with/ without consolidation) and are non-rounded/non-peripheral. • Limited GGO with a non-peripheral distribution and non-rounded.	"Imaging aspects can be seen with pneumonia."
Atypical structure/ appearance	Uncommonly or not stated aspects of COVID-19 pneumonia.	• Nonappearance of indeterminate or typical aspects AND appearance of segmental consolidation without GGO. • Discrete minor nodules. • Lung cavitation • Smooth interlobular septal thickening with pleural effusion	"Imaging aspects are unusually stated for pneumonia. Alternative analyses can be considered."
Negative (-ve) for pneumonia	No aspects of pneumonia	None of the CT aspects recommended to pneumonia	None of the CT results available to specify pneumonia(Note:- CT can be negative (-ve) in the early stages of COVID-19.)."

transmission even after clinical recovery. The highest transmission risk of COVID-19 is between healthcare workers. The number of COVID-19-infected people around the world is increasing, as is the death rate. The doctor who first warned about the COVID-19 virus has also died. Hence, there is need a to prevent COVID-19 virus transmission.

TABLE 2.3

Non-pulmonary organs affected by COVID-19

	Complications	Symptoms
Cardiovascular	Myocardial injury, heart failure, pulmonary embolism, deep vein thrombosis, demand ischemia, myocarditis,	Shortness of breath, chest pain, hemoptysis
Neurological	Acute hemorrhagic necrotizing encephalopathy, acute cerebrovascular disease	Impaired consciousness, central nervous system(CNS) –ataxia, headache, acute cerebrovascular disease, dizziness, skeletal muscular symptoms (neuralgia, hypogeusia and hyposmia), and peripheralnervous system(PNS) symptoms
Abdominal	Alkalosis, acute renal injury, hyperkalemia, abnormal liver function tests	Vomiting, abdominal pain, nausea, diarrhea
Hematological	Lymphocytopenia, thrombocytosis, leukocytosis, hemophagocytic lymphohistocytosis, disseminated intravascular coagulation	
Musculoskeletal	Rhabdomyolysis	Myalgia

These prevention steps need to be followed:

- Suspected or confirmed cases should isolate at home and undergo continued testing with sampling intervals.
- Good ventilation and sunlight damage the virus. Generally, the negative pressure room is not recommended.
- Hands should be washed often with hand sanitizer or soap and water.
- Patients must wear surgical masks.
- Caretakers must wear surgical masks indoors and sanitatise hands every 15–20 minutes.
- Maintain at least one metre's distance from other people (market places, offices, hospitals, medical stores etc.).
- Surfaces, rooms and equipment must be sanitised regularly.
- Avoid frequent trips to outside places (market places, medical supplies etc.).
- Avoid hand shaking and hugging as a means of greeting.
- Avoid social gatherings at home.
- Don't allow visitors at home.
- Healthcare workers should be provided with N95 masks, protective suits and goggles.

The Ministry of Health and Family Welfare of the Government of India has declared these steps should be followed to avoid spreading COVID-19:

- Wash hands often with hand sanitizer or soap and water.
- Use mask to cover mouth and nose.
- Cover nose and mouth while sneezing and coughing.
- Socially distance.
- Clean and disinfect frequently-touched surfaces daily.

The virus spreads from one person to another through respiratory droplets from an infected person's cough or sneeze.

2.5   DISCUSSION

The quick epidemic of COVID-19 is a new virus infection first reported in Wuhan City, China. The primary symptoms for this virus are respiratory problems, fever, cold, cough, and so on. Therefore, various authors have recommended chest CT for initial and severe stages (Bernheim et al., 2020; Awulachew et al., 2020; Chung et al., 2020). According to the report, specificity of chest CT in identifying COVID-19 is higher than RT-PCR testing. Using chest CT, the author achieved an accuracy rate of 94% in analysing COVID-19 imaging features, as reported in the current meta-analysis (Kim et al., 2020b). CT scans should be done within the first two days of symptoms, and the results are usually determined by RT-PCR. Based on analysis of chest CT in the initial stage, it is more effective than RT-PCR among hospitalized patients. With signs of fever and respiratory tract within 14 days, the suspicion of COVID-19 is too strong in an effective clinical environment. Suspected cases of COVID-19 in the first 14 days need common laboratory findings, namely, elevated inflammatory markers, lymphopenia, elevated liver enzymes, and so on. In this situation, RT-PCR is recommended by Chendrasekhar (2020) since it is the gold standard for identifying COVID-19. Some of the drawbacks of RT-PCR include the sensitivity of COVID-19, availability, and increased waiting times in the results portion; additionally, can affect the quality samples in RT-PCR. Finally it is concluded that, RT-PCR is potentially effective but has some resource limitations (Chendrasekhar, 2020). One of the authors has applied correlation among the results of CT scans and RT-PCR (Ai et al., 2020). It has higher Positive Predictive Value (PPV) and accuracy of chest CT scan in patients younger than 60. In patients younger than 50 years, however, the author discovered a significantly lower sensitivity and a significantly higher specificity. This result has been explained in a high amount of CT scans without any mediastinal or parenchymal alteration in the younger group. This is because the patients are affected by heart failure. The low percentage of RT-PCR rates with less than 50 patients showed high specificity, as analysed by Leeflang et al. (2013). In a recent review Raptis et al. (2020) mentions study (Bai et al., 2020) reported high CT specificity and they accepted as genuine report in a clinical applications. Various research has been conducted and reported about association of chest-CT and image findings of COVID-19 (Simpson et al., 2020: Chung et al., 2020). The same literature has been encountered with CT symptoms of Congestive Heart Failure (CSF) and pulmonary edoema, which mostly overlaps with COVID-19 pneumonia. In this case, radiologists must be very careful in diagnosing SARS-CoV-2. COVID-19 is evaluated by low dose high resolution CT scans protocol and achieved 89% sensitivity and 85% specificity (Radpour et al. 2020). These results support the use of imaging features to diagnose COVID-19. Therefore, the review report recommends chest CT as a cost-effective and rapid screening tool to analyse the imaging features of COVID-19 patients. According to the report, the SARS-CoV-2 viral load becomes very complex. This chapter has given a review report on various modalities considered for COVID-19 and shown their performances. From the performance analysis, it is evident that chest CT is highly recommended over other modalities due to its high quality, sensitivity and speed. Several studies have reported that Chest CT can serve as a superior diagnosis tool to other screening modalities.

2.6 CONCLUSION

COVID-19, with a severe pathology, is a group of single-stranded and enveloped RNA viruses. An analysis of the imaging features of COVID-19 using multi-modalities, namely, MRI, CT, PET/CT, US and CXR, has been conducted in this study. The features are investigated and imaging findings of COVID-19 for all the modalities are revealed. These imaging features help in early detection of SARS-CoV-2 and MERS. Mixed attenuation opacities and multilobar, mainly peripheral and basilar ground-glass are the most common imaging findings, according to CXR and CT observations. In the identification of slight pulmonary changes, CXR provides poor sensitivity for mild or early stages of the disease, but it can be helpful in monitoring care and triaging patients with radiographically-demonstrable pneumonia. The changes in CT are used to explain a pattern of temporal evolution and pneumonia as a response to acute lung injury. POC evaluation in Chest CT has been useful, and the CT findings are highly correlated. Similarly, the PET/CT and MRI findings have been comprehensively defined; the PET/CT and MRI images prove that they are closely related to the characteristics of CT imaging presence. RT-PCR is now viewed as the gold standard for COVID-19 detection. Chest CT is a quicker alternative, and sensitive to RT-PCR in diagnosing COVID-19 for hospitalized patients. Among all the modalities, CT findings proved the best screening method of COVID-19 patients, compared to other modalities. Finally this work concluded that, CT is giving more support to radiologists and service providers to analyse and diagnose COVID-19. This leads the doctors to proceed further.

REFERENCES

Ai, T., Yang, Z., Hou, H., Zhan, C., Chen, C., Lv, W., & Xia, L. (2020). Correlation of chest CT and RT-PCR testing in coronavirus disease 2019 (COVID-19) in China: a report of 1014 cases. *Radiology*, 1: 1–23. https://doi.org/10.1148/radiol.2020200642.

Awulachew, E., Diriba, K., Anja, A., Getu, E., & Belayneh, F. (2020). Computed tomography (CT) imaging features of patients with COVID-19: systematic review and meta-analysis. *Radiology Research and Practice*. https://doi.org/10.1155/2020/1023506.

Bai, H. X., Hsieh, B., Xiong, Z., Halsey, K., Choi, J. W., Tran, T. M. L., & Liao, W. H. (2020). Performance of radiologists in differentiating COVID-19 from non-COVID-19 viral pneumonia at chest CT. *Radiology*. https://doi.org/10.1148/radiol.2020200823.

Bernheim A., Mei X., Huang M., Yang, Y., Fayad, Z. A., Zhang, N., & Chung, M. (2020). Chest CT findings in coronavirus disease-19 (COVID-19): relationship to duration of infection. *Radiology*. doi: 10.1148/radiol.2020200463.

Buonsenso, D., Piano, A., Raffaelli, F., Bonadia, N., de Gaetano Donati, K., Franceschi, F. (2020). Point-of-care lung ultrasound findings in novel coronavirus disease-19 pneumoniae: a case report and potential applications during COVID-19 outbreak. *European Review for Medical and Pharmacological Science*, 24:2776–2780.

Chan, J. F. W., Yuan, S., Kok, K.-H., Kai-Wang, K., Chu, H., Yang, J., & Yuen, K.-Y. (2020). A familial cluster of pneumonia associated with the 2019 novel coronavirus indicating person-to-person transmission: a study of a family cluster. *The Lancet*. https://doi.org/10.1016/S0140-6736(20)30154-9.

Chaplin, S. (2020). COVID-19: a brief history and treatments in development. *Prescriber*. https://doi.org/10.1002/psb.1843.

Chauhan, S. (2020). Comprehensive review of coronavirus disease 2019 (COVID-19). *Biomedical Journal*. https://doi.org/10.1016/j.bj.2020.05.023.

Chen, N., Zhou, M., Dong, X., Qu, J., Gong, F., Han, Y., & Zhang, L. (2020). Epidemiological and clinical characteristics of 99 cases of 2019 novel coronavirus pneumonia in Wuhan, China: a descriptive study. *The Lancet*, 395(10226):809–815.

Chen, H., Guo, J., Wang, C., Luo, F., Yu, X., Zhang, W., & Zhang, Y. (2020). Clinical characteristics and intrauterine vertical transmission potential of COVID-19 infection in nine pregnant women: a retrospective review of medical records. *Lancet*. https://doi.org/10.1016/S0140-6736(20)30360-3.

Chendrasekhar, A. (2020). Chest CT versus RT-PCR for diagnostic accuracy of COVID-19 detection: a meta-analysis. *Journal of Vascular Medicine & Surgery*, 8(3):1–4.

Cheng Z. J., Shan J. (2019). Novel coronavirus: where we are and what we know. *Infection*, 2020:1–9. https://doi.org/10.1007/s15010-020-01401-y.

Cheng, Z. J., Shan, J. (2020). 2019 novel coronavirus: where we are and what we know. *Infection*, 48(2): 155–163.

Chung, M. et al. 2020. "CT Imaging Features of 2019 Novel Coronavirus (2019-NCoV)." *Radiology*. https://doi.org/10.1148/radiol.2020200230.

Chung, M., Bernheim, A., Mei, X., Zhang, N., Huang, M., Zheng, X., & Shan, H. (2020). CT imaging features of 2019 novel coronavirus (2019-nCoV). *Radiology*, 295(1):202–207, https://doi.org/10.1148/radiol.2020200230.

Copetti, R. (2016). Is lung ultrasound the stethoscope of the new millennium? Definitely yes! Acta Medica Academica. https://doi.org/10.5644/ama2006-124.162.

Corman, V. M., Landt, O., Kaiser, A., Molenkamp, R., Meijer, A., Chu, D. K. W., & Drosten, C. (2020). Detection of 2019 Novel Coronavirus (2019-NCoV) by Real-Time RT-PCR. *Eurosurveillance*.

Coronavirus Outbreak. 2020. Available at: https://www.worldometers.info/coronavirus/.

Czawlytko, C., Hossain, R., & White, C. S. (2020). COVID-19 diagnostic imaging recommendations. *Applied Radiology*, 49(3): 10–15.

Das, K. M., Lee, E. Y., Singh, R., Enani, M. A., Dossari, K. A., Gorkom, K. V., & Langer, R. D. (2017). Follow-up chest radiographic findings in patients with MERS-CoV after recovery. *Indian Journal of Radiology* and Imaging, 27(3):342–349.

Das Karuna, M., Lee, E. Y., Langer, R. D., and Larsson, S. G. (2016). Middle East respiratory syndrome coronavirus: what does a radiologist need to know? *American Journal of Roentgenology*, 206(6):1193–1201.

De Souza, L., Kleber, L., Heiser, V., Regamey, N., Panning, M., Drexler, J. F., & Drosten, C. (2007). Generic detection of coronaviruses and differentiation at the prototype strain level by reverse transcription-PCR and nonfluorescent low-density microarray. *Journal of Clinical Microbiology*, 45(3):1049–1052.

Dhama, K., Khan, S., Tiwari, R., Sircar, S., Bhat, S., Malik, Y. S., & Alfonso (2020). Coronavirus disease 2019-COVID-19, clinical microbiology reviews. *American Society of Microbiology*, 1:4–48.

Dos, S., Gouvea, W. (2020). Natural history of COVID-19 and current knowledge on treatment therapeutic options. *Biomedicine and Pharmacotherapy*, 29(1):1–1 8.

Dos Santos, W. G. (2020). Natural history of COVID-19 and current knowledge on treatment therapeutic options. *Biomedicine and Pharmacotherapy*. https://doi.org/10.1016/j.biopha.2020.110493.

Falaschi, Zeno, Danna, P. S. C., Arioli, R., Pasché, A., Zagaria, D., Percivale, I., & Carriero, A. (2020). Chest CT accuracy in diagnosing COVID-19 during the peak of the Italian Epidemic: a retrospective correlation with RT-PCR testing and analysis of discordant cases. *European Journal of Radiology*.

Fan Y., Zhao K., Shi Z. L., Zhou P. 2019. Bat coronaviruses in China. *Viruses* 11:210. https://doi.org/10.3390/v11030210.

Fang, Y., Zhang, H., Xie, J., Lin, M., Ying, L., Pang, P., & Ji, W. (2020). Sensitivity of chest CT for COVID-19: Comparison to RT-PCR. *Radiology*. https://doi.org/10.1148/radiol.2020200432.

Giannitto, C., Sposta, F. M., Repici, A., Vatteroni, G., Casiraghi, E., Casari, E., & Luca, B. (2020). Chest CT in patients with a moderate or high pretest probability of COVID-19 and negative swab. *Radiologia Medica*. https://doi.org/10.1007/s11547-020-01269-w.

Gralinski, L. E., and Vineet, D. M. (2020). Return of the coronavirus: 2019-NCoV. *Viruses*, 12:135. https://doi.org/10.3390/v12020135.

Guan, C. S., Lv, Z. B., Yan, S., Du, Y. N., Chen, H., Wei, L. G., & Chen, B. D. (2020a, May). Imaging features of coronavirus disease 2019 (COVID-19): evaluation on thin-section CT. *Academic Radiology*. 27(5):609–613. doi: 10.1016/j.acra.2020.03.002. Epub 2020 Mar 20. PMID: 32204990; PMCID: PMC7156158.

Guan, W., Ni, Z., Hu, Y., Liang, W., Ou, C., He, J., & Zhong, N. (2020b). Clinical characteristics of coronavirus disease 2019 in China. *New England Journal of Medicine*. https://doi.org/10.1056/nejmoa2002032.

Hageman, J. R. (2020). The coronavirus disease 2019 (COVID-19). *Pediatric Annals*, 49(3): e99–e100.

Hansell, D. M., Bankier, A. A., Macmahon, H., McLoud, T. C., Müller, N. L., & Remy, J. (2008). Fleischner society: Glossary of terms for thoracic imaging. *Radiology*. https://doi.org/10.1148/radiol.2462070712.

Hosseiny, M., Kooraki, S., Gholamrezanezhad, A., Reddy, S., and Myers, L. (2020). *Radiology* perspective of coronavirus disease 2019 (COVID-19): lessons from severe acute respiratory syndrome and middle east respiratory syndrome, *American Journal of Roentgenology*, 214(5):1078–1082.

Huang, C., Wang, Y., Li, X., Ren, L., Zhao, J., Hu, Y., & Cao, B. (2020). Clinical features of patients infected with 2019 novel coronavirus in Wuhan, China. *The Lancet*. https://doi.org/10.1016/S0140-6736(20)30183-5.

Jin, Y. H., Cai, L., Cheng, Z. S., Cheng, H., Deng, T., Fan, Y. P., & Wang, X. H. (2020). A rapid advice guideline for the diagnosis and treatment of 2019 novel coronavirus (2019-NCoV) infected pneumonia (standard version). *Military Medical Research*. https://doi.org/10.1186/s40779-020-0233-6.

Johnson, N. P. A. S., and Mueller, J. (2002). Updating the accounts: global mortality of the 1918-1920 'Spanish' influenza pandemic. *Bulletin of the History of Medicine*. https://doi.org/10.1353/bhm.2002.0022.

Kain, T., and Fowler, R. (2019). Preparing intensive care for the next pandemic influenza. *Critical Care*, 23(1):1–9.

Ketai, L., Paul, N. S., Wong, K. T. (2006). Radiology of severe acute respiratory syndrome (SARS): the emerging pathologic-radiologic correlates of an emerging disease. *Journal of Thoracic Imaging*, 21:276–283.

Kim, H., Hong, H., & Ho Yoon, S. (2020a). Diagnostic performance of ct and reverse transcriptase polymerase chain reaction for coronavirus disease 2019: a meta-analysis. *Radiology*. https://doi.org/10.1148/radiol.2020201343.

Kim, J. Y., Choe, P. G., Oh, Y., Kim, J., Park, S. J., Park, J. H., & Oh, M. D. (2020b). The first case of 2019 novel coronavirus pneumonia imported into Korea from Wuhan, China: implication for infection prevention and control measures. *Journal of Korean Medical Science*. https://doi.org/10.3346/jkms.2020.35.e61.

Kumar, D (2020). Coronavirus: a review of COVID-19. *Eurasian Journal of Medicine and Oncology*, 4(1):8–25.

Leeflang, M. M. G., Rutjes, A. W. S., Reitsma, J. B., Hooft, L., & Bossuyt, P. M. M. (2013). Variation of a test's sensitivity and specificity with disease prevalence. *CMAJ*. https://doi.org/10.1503/cmaj.121286.

Letko, M., Marzi, A., and Munster V. (2020). Functional assessment of cell entry and receptor usage for SARS-CoV-2 and other lineage B betacoronaviruses. *Nature Microbiology*.

Li, Q., Guan, X., Wu, P., Wang, X., Zhou, L., Tong, Y., & Feng, Z. (2020). Early transmission dynamics in Wuhan, China, of novel Coronavirus–infected pneumonia. *New England Journal of Medicine*. https://doi.org/10.1056/nejmoa2001316.

Liu, Y., Chin, R. L., Kuo, and Shih, S. R. (2020). COVID-19: the first documented coronavirus pandemic in history. *Biomedical Journal*. https://doi.org/10.1016/j.bj.2020.04.007.

Lu, R., Zhao, X., Li, J., Niu, P., Yang, B., Wu, H., & Tan, W. (2020). Genomic characterisation and epidemiology of 2019 novel coronavirus: implications for virus origins and receptor binding. *Lancet*, 395:565.

Manna, S., Wruble, J., Maron, S. Z., Toussie, D., Voutsinas, N., Finkelstein, M., & Bernheim, A. (2020). COVID-19: a multimodality review of radiologic techniques, clinical utility, and imaging features. *Radiology*: Cardiothoracic Imaging. https://doi.org/10.1148/ryct.2020200210.

Peng, Q. Y., Wang, X. T., & Zhang, L. N. (2020). Findings of lung ultrasonography of novel coronavirus pneumonia during the 2019–2020 epidemic. *Intensive Care Medicine*. https://doi.org/10.1007/s00134-020-05996-6.

Pyrc, K., Berkhout, B., and van der Hoek, L. (2007). The novel human coronaviruses NL63 and HKU1. *Journal of Virology*.

Radpour, A., Bahrami-Motlagh, H., Taaghi, M. T., Sedaghat, A., Karimi, M. A., Hekmatnia, A., & Azhideh, A. (2020). COVID-19 evaluation by low-dose high resolution CT scans protocol. *Academic Radiology*. https://doi.org/10.1016/j.acra.2020.04.016.

Raptis, C. A., Hammer, M. M., Short, R. G., Henry, T. S., Hope, M. D., Bhalla, S. (2020). Chest CT and coronavirus disease (COVID-19): a critical review of the literature to date, [published online ahead of print, 2020 Apr 16], *AJR American Journal of Roentgenoogy*, l. 1–4, https://doi.org/10.2214/ AJR.20.23202.

Sheng, W. H. (2020). Coronavirus disease 2019 (COVID-19). *Journal of Internal Medicine of Taiwan*, 31(2):61–66.

Shi, H., Han, X., Jiang, N., Cao, Y., Alwalid, O., Gu, J., & Zheng, C. (2020). Radiological findings from 81 patients with COVID-19 pneumonia in Wuhan, China: a descriptive study. *The Lancet Infectious Diseases*. https://doi.org/10.1016/S1473-3099(20)30086-4.

Simonsen, L., Clarke, M. J., Schonberger, S. B., Arden, N. H., Cox, N. J., Fakuda, K. (1998). Pandemic versus epidemic influenza mortality: a pattern of changing age distribution. *Journal of Infectious Diseases*. https://doi.org/10.1086/515616.

Simpson, S., Kay, F. U., Abbara, S., Bhalla, S., Chung, J. H., Chung, M., Litt, H. (2020). Radiological Society of North America Expert Consensus Statement on Reporting

Chest CT Findings Related to COVID-19. Endorsed by the Society of Thoracic Radiology, the American College of Radiology, and RSNA. *Radiology: Cardiothoracic Imaging*. https://doi.org/10.1148/ryct.2020200152.

Singhal, T. (2020). A review of coronavirus disease-2019 (COVID-19) *Indian Journal of Pediatrics*, 87(4):281–286.

Sun, P., Lu, X., Xu, C., Sun, W., and Pan, B. (2020). Understanding of COVID-19 based on current evidence. *Journal of Medical Virology*. https://doi.org/10.1002/jmv.25722.

World Health Organization. 2020. A & A practice coronavirus disease (COVID-19) Situation Report – 198.

World Health Organization. Situation reports. Available at: https:// www.who.int/emergencies/ diseases/novel-coronavirus-2019/situation-reports/. Accessed 22 Feb 2020.

Xiong, Y., Zhang, Q., Zhao, L., Shao, J., Zhu, W. (2020). Clinical and imaging features of COVID-19 in a Neonate. *Chest*. https://doi.org/10.1016/j.chest.2020.03.018.

Yang, Y., Yang, M., Shen, C., Wang, F., Yuan, J., Li, J., & Liu, Y. (2020). Laboratory diagnosis and monitoring the viral shedding of 2019-nCoV infections. *MedRxiv*, 1(3):1–6.

Zhu, N., Zhang, D., Wang, W., Li, X., Yang, B., Song, J., & Tan, W. (2020). A novel coronavirus from patients with pneumonia in China, 2019. *New England Journal of Medicine*. https://doi.org/10.1056/nejmoa2001017.

Zou, S. and Zhu, X. (2020). FDG PET/CT of COVID-19. *Radiology*. 200770.

Zu, Z., Jiang, M., Xu, P., Chen, W., Ni, Q. Q., Lu, G. M., Zhang, L. J. (2020). Coronavirus disease 2019 (COVID-19): a perspective from China. *Radiology*. 200490. doi:10.1148/ radiol.2020200490.

3 Investigation of COVID-19 Chest X-ray Images using Texture Features – A Comprehensive Approach

J. Thamil Selvi, K. Subhashini, and M. Methini
Department of ECE, Sri Sairam Engineering College, Chennai, India

3.1 INTRODUCTION

COVID-19 is an infectious disease which affects the respiratory system. It is a type of pneumonia, which is most challenging to nternational health [Salehi et al., 2020]. Coronaviruses are the largest ever discovered, enveloped with single-stranded, positive sense RNA genome and identified as new zootomic human coronaviruses (HCoV) of the century [Zhu et al., 2020, Su et al., 2016]. It emerged as a worldwide epidemic and the World Health Organization (WHO) declared it as a pandemic called COVID-19 [Iqbal et al., 2020, Siddiqui et al., 2020]. WHO reported more than 8.86 million positive cases and about 465,000 deaths due to COVID-19 [WHO, 2020]. The mortality rate increases due to Acute Respiratory Distress Syndrome (ARDS) or pulmonary embolism [Parry and Wani, 2020]. To reduce the mortality and morbidity rate early, diagnosis is crucial.

Reverse transcription polymerase chain reaction (RT-PCR) is a screening method to diagnose COVID-19 [Wang et al., 2020]. The positive rate is only 30% to 60%, so it fails to control the spread of contiguous diseases [Yang et al., 2020]. To reduce false negatives, automated analysis is necessary. Chest X-ray imaging is a common, easy and fast tool for pneumonia diagnosis. X-ray images show visual indexes correlated with COVID-19 [Kanne et al., 2020]. Basu and Mitra (2020) attempted Domain Extension Transfer Learning. In this technique, significant features of chest X-ray images were extracted and applied to classification. ConvNet model was attempted to classify the X-ray images [Kermany et al., 2018]. Literature also reported that data mining techniques were attempted to identify SARS and pneumonia from x-ray images [Xie et al., 2006]. COVID-19 was also diagnosed by analyzing the alveolar opacities of chest X-rays [Kim et al., 2020]. Sun et al. (2020)

45

studied the homogeneity of corona-positive and corona-negative CT images using a Chi-square test. Deep-learning models, such as DenseNet-121 and Dense Net-RNN, were used to identify pneumonia [Li et al. 2018]. In this study, chest X-rays were used for analysis. A deep-learning-based AI system was implemented to differentiate COVID-19 patients [Murphy et al., 2020]; results were validated by six independent readers. To classify COVID-19 patients, a subjective study using chest X-ray was performed by a Radiologist [Cozzi et al., 2020]; statistical analysis was reported using Excel. A decision tree model of X-ray and CT scan images used Convolution Neural Networks(CNN) [Dansana et al., 2020]. Silva et al. (2020) developed an efficient CovidNet framework to detect COVID-19 patterns in CT images. Due to insufficient images, accuracy was minimal.

Many reviews in the literature report invasive methods, such as swab and PCR tests, and non-invasive methods, such as Artificial intelligence and deep-learning, in screening for COVID-19. In this work an attempt is made to investigate COVID-19 X-ray images using textural features. First order, second order and higher order statistical features are extracted from normal and abnormal chest X-rays. The extracted features are analyzed to find significant ones, which could classify normal and abnormal images.

3.2 METHODOLOGY

3.2.1 DATABASE

Chest X-ray images for this study are obtained from online the database https://www.kaggle.com/datasets. 25 normal images and 25 COVID-19-positive (abnormal) images were obtained. Texture features were extracted and investigated.

3.2.2 MATERIALS AND METHODS

To investigate normal and abnormal chest X-ray images, texture features are extracted and analyzed. Texture is vital descriptor of an image. Textural features capture spatial arrangement of gray values. Based on the number of pixels, the statistical feature can be of first, second or higher order.

First-order statistical features are extracted directly from pixel intensity. They do not consider the relationship of pixels with neighboring pixels. Mean, median, mode, kurtosis and skewness are first-order features extracted from normal and abnormal images [Han et al., 2013].

Gray Level Difference Statistics (GLDS) [Srinivasan and Shobha, 2008] are used for texture analysis. They consider local properties based on the absolute difference in pixel intensity. Features such as contrast, energy, entropy and mean are obtained by summing the single gray level difference probability distribution vector at four different angles: 0; 45; 90; and 135 degrees. Contrast quantifies overall variation in image intensity and measures the intensity of neighboring pixels over the entire image. Increased contrast reflects a heterogeneous texture pattern. Energy is the measure of uniformity among the pixels. Entropy measures the distribution of gray values.

$$s_i = \left\{ \sum_{p \in N_i} i - M_p \right\} \tag{3.1}$$

Using the matrix, features such as coarseness, contrast, strength, busyness and complexity are extracted from the Neighborhood Gray Tone Difference method (NGTDM). From the normal and abnormal images, these features are extracted and analyzed.

Coarseness measures the roughness of the surface components of the large particles it is composed of. It is expressed using equation (3.2)

$$f_{coars} = \left[\varepsilon + \sum_{i=0}^{G_h} p_i s_i \right]^{-1} \tag{3.2}$$

P_i = probability of occurrence of gray values

G_h = the largest gray tone

ε = small value to cope with the division and S_i is a matrix obtained from (3.1).

Intensity, the difference between neighboring regions, reflects contrast and is expressed by equation (3.3)

$$f_{con} = \left[\frac{1}{N_g(N_g - 1)} \sum_{i=0}^{G_h} \sum_{j=0}^{G_h} p_i p_j (i - j)^2 \right] \left[\frac{1}{n} \sum_{i=0}^{G_h} s(i) \right] \tag{3.3}$$

$$N_g = \sum_{i=0}^{G_h} Q_i$$

N_g is the summation of different gray-tones present in the image

Q_i = 1 if $p_i \neq 0$; else, the value is zero.

The spatial frequency of intensity changes are calculated using equation (3.4) which is known as busyness.

$$\frac{\sum_{i=0}^{G_h} p_i s_i}{\sum_{i=0}^{G_h} \sum_{j=0}^{G_h} ip_i - jp_j} \tag{3.4}$$

where p_i, $p_j \neq 0$

Complexity depicts high information when the patches such as texture of the images are heterogeneous.

Texture strength is the ratio of intensity difference between adjacent primitives, which depends on the probability of occurrences and sum of deviation from the centre pixel with respect to surrounding pixels.

Chest X-ray images are filtered using LAWS mask. Texture energy is computed from the filtered image by summing the absolute values of pixels and their neighborhood. Three filters with corresponding masks, such as L-averaging filter [1 4 6 4 1], E-Edge detector filter [-1 -2 0 2 1] and S- Spot detector filter [-1 0 2 0 -1] [Rachidi et al., 2008] are used and convolved with each other to create 5 × 5 2D mask kernel LL, EE, LE, ES and LS. These masks are applied over an image to obtain a filtered image. The energy from filtered images is extracted using

$$TEM(x, y) = \sum_{(u,v) \in S_r(x,y)} |filtered\_image(u, v)| \qquad (3.5)$$

where $(u, v) \in S_r(x, y) \leftrightarrow \sqrt{(u - x)^2 + (v - y)^2} \leq r$, $S_r(x, y)$ is the neighborhood of (x, y) at radius 'r'.

The extracted features are used to analyze normal and pathological subjects.

The Statistical Feature Matrix (SFM) extracts visual texture features by considering the intersample spacing between the pixels [Loizou et al., 2015]. Features such as Coarseness, Contrast, Periodicity and Roughness are extracted from normal and abnormal chest X-ray images, then extracted and analysed.

Higher order texture features are extracted by constructing a Gray Level Run Length (GLRL) Matrix [Galloway and Mm (1975)]. Gray level run and run length are defined as consecutive pixels with similar intensities and number of pixel in a run. To extract textural features from the images gray level run matrix are computed in 0, 45, 90 and 135 degree direction. The elements in the run length matrix are: G is the number of gray levels; R is the run; and N is the number or pixels in the image. Some of the features extracted from GLRL matrix are represented by the equation. In GLRL features, the similarity of gray levels are measured using Gray Level Nonuniformity (GLN) and is given by

$$GLN = \frac{\sum_{i=1}^{G} \left(\sum_{j=1}^{R} p(i, j) | \theta \right)^2}{\sum_{i=1}^{G} \sum_{j=1}^{R} p(i, j) | \theta} \qquad (3.6)$$

The similarity of the length of the runs is measured using Run Length Nonuniformity (RLN), and Run Percentage (RP), which measures the homogeneity and distribution of runs at specific direction and is given by

$$RLN = \frac{\sum_{j=1}^{G} \left(\sum_{i=1}^{R} p(i, j) | \theta \right)^2}{\sum_{i=1}^{G} \sum_{j=1}^{R} p(i, j) | \theta} \qquad (3.7)$$

$$RP = \frac{1}{N} \sum_{i=1}^{G} \sum_{j=1}^{R} p(i, j) | \theta \qquad (3.8)$$

Similarly high gray level run emphasis (HGRE) is found to be large when pixel intensity is high, which is given by

$$HGRE = \frac{\sum_{i=1}^{G} \sum_{j=1}^{R} i^2 p(i, j) | \theta}{\sum_{i=1}^{G} \sum_{j=1}^{R} p(i, j) | \theta} \qquad (3.9)$$

Another feature extraction functions using joint statistical measures of gray level and run length described in [Dasarathy and Holder (1991)] was attempted and extracted. The larger values of Short Run Low Gray Level Emphasis (SRLGE) are observed in the images for short runs with low pixel intensity.

$$SRLGE = \frac{\sum_{i=1}^{G} \sum_{j=1}^{R} \frac{p(i,j)\,|\,\theta}{i^2 j^2}}{\sum_{i=1}^{G} \sum_{j=1}^{R} p(i,j)|\theta} \qquad (3.10)$$

3.3 RESULTS AND DISCUSSION

Typical gray scale chest X-ray images are shown in Figure 3.1. Normal image with clear rib cage is shown in Figure 3.1a. A Corona-positive chest X-ray, or abnormal, is shown in Figure 3.1b. A total of 25 normal and abnormal images are considered for this study. From the normal and abnormal images, five first-order statistical features, 23 GLCM features, four GLDS, four SFM, five NGTDM, six LAWS texture measure features and 11 GLRL features are extracted and analyzed.

First-order features are obtained by considering pixel intensity only. From the normal and abnormal images, researchers extracted five first-order statistical features: mean; median; mode; skewness; and kurtosis. These are shown in Figure 3.2. Mode is found to be high in normal images as compared to abnormal images. This may be due to occurrence of uniform pixel intensity in the normal image. Skewness and kurtosis are observed to be high in abnormal images, which may be due to lack of symmetry in pixel intensity in the pathological condition. The high value of mean and median in normal images depicts increased pixel intensity.

First-order statistical features are obtained directly from the pixel intensity without considering the spatial relationship among pixels. Hence, features extracted by considering spatial relationships of pixels in normal and abnormal images are analyzed by constructing the gray-level co-occurrence matrix (GLCM). The mean and standard deviation of the statistical features extracted from the GLCM are tabulated in the Table 3.1.

(a)   (b)

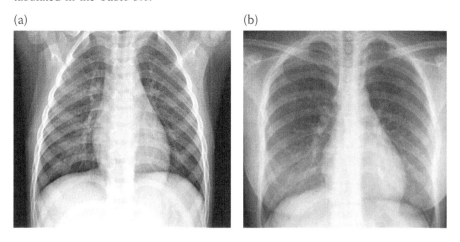

FIGURE 3.1 Typical chest X-ray images: (a) Normal (b) Corona positive (abnormal).

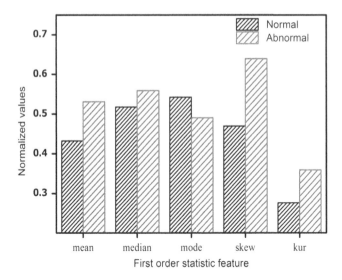

FIGURE 3.2 First-order statistical feature.

To extract significant features from the normal and abnormal images, a student t-test was performed. Among 23 GLCM features, six features - autocorrelation, contrast, dissimilarity, energy, entropy and homogeneity - were observed to be significant, with a correlation of $p < 0.05$. A box plot was constructed and is shown in Figure 3.3.

From Figure 3.3 it is clear that the box plot could distinguish normal from abnormal features. Contrast and entropy are efficient in differentiating normal and abnormal features by 22%. It shows the range of abnormal features is high, which may be due to a pathological condition or increased pixel intensity.

Gray level difference statistics is based on the differences among gray levels. Four features are extracted from normal and abnormal images, as shown in Figure 3.4. It is observed that mean and contrast values are found to be high in

TABLE 3.1

Normalized mean and standard deviation of GLCM feature

Features	Mean ± Std dev	
	Normal Images	Abnormal Images
Autocorrelation	0.44 ± 0.25	0.52 ± 0.26
Contrast	0.38 ± 0.21	0.59 ± 0.29
Dissimilarity	0.38 ± 0.22	0.43 ± 0.27
Energy	0.50 ± 0.34	0.32 ± 0.33
Entropy	0.41 ± 0.31	0.63 ± 0.31
Homogeneity	0.62 ± 0.22	0.59 ± 0.29

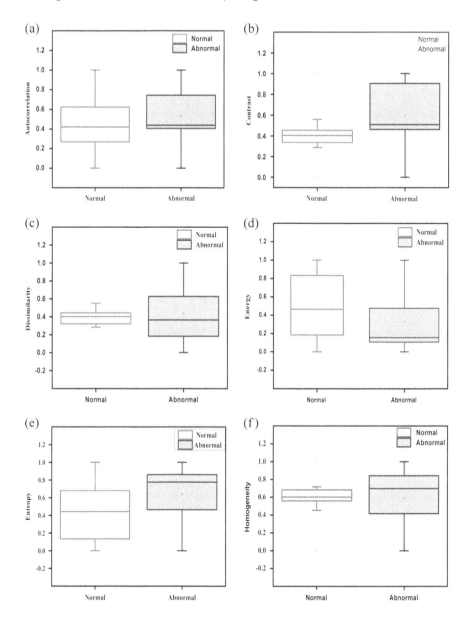

FIGURE 3.3 Box plot representation of statitically-significant GLCM features: (a) Autocorrelation (b) Contrast (c) Dissimilarity (d) Energy (e) Entropy and (f) Homogeneity.

abnormal images. This may be due to large edge magnitude and variations in pixel intensity. Due to randomness of intensity variation in abnormal images, entropy is observed to be high. Normal images tend to have a uniform intensity value, which leads to increased energy.

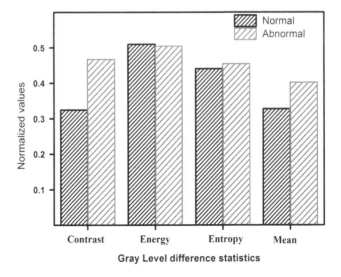

FIGURE 3.4   Gray level difference statistics feature.

The statistical features based on interpixel spatial distance – coarseness, periodicity, roughness and contrast – are extracted from normal and pathological images, as shown in Figure 3.5. Abnormal images display high contrast, which may be due to a sudden increase in pixel intensity of pathological subjects. Periodicity, roughness and coarseness are observed to be high in normal images. This may be because there is less difference in pixel value with respect to adjacent pixels, or due to smooth repetitive patterns among the pixels. A high roughness value is observed

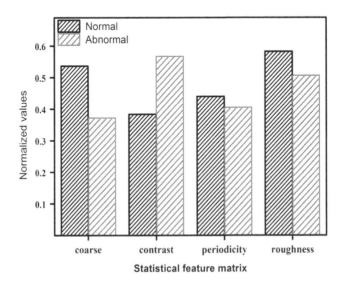

FIGURE 3.5   Statistical Feature Matrix.

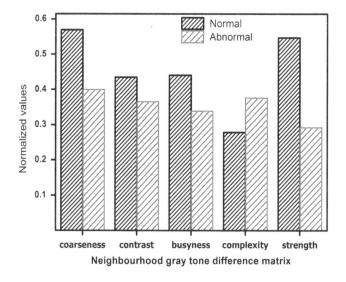

FIGURE 3.6 Neighborhood gray tone difference matrix.

in normal images due to similar intensity values in the neighborhood. Among the features, contrast differed between normal and abnormal images by 18%.

Features extracted from the neighborhood gray tone difference matrix are shown in Figure 3.6. Among the observed features, complexity is found to be high in abnormal images. This may be due to the presence of pixel primitives with varying average intensities. Due to an increase in probability of occurrence of pixel intensity, the strength of normal images is observed to be high. Coarseness, contrast and busyness are high in normal, compared with abnormal, images. The busyness of

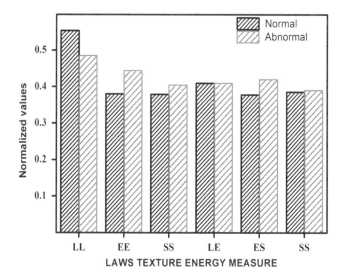

FIGURE 3.7 LAWS texture feature.

normal images is high due to spatial frequency intensity changes. As the intensity variation between the pixels of normal images is high, this in turn results in high contrast. Coarseness, strength and busyness show distinct variation between normal and abnormal subjects. Among the features, strength demarcated normal and abnormal images by 27%.

Texture energy extracted using Laws mask from normal and abnormal chest X-rays is shown in Figure 3.7. Energy is the feature which reflects uniformity among the pixels. Figure 3.4 shows TEM among normal and abnormal images. It is observed that in almost all the kernels, energy is high in abnormal images due to absence of repeated pairs of pixels. An abnormal image with high energy implies significant variation in the texture, due to variation in pixel intensities. In the LL kernel, a normal image is observed with high energy. This may be due to texture uniformity among the gray levels, and repeated pairs of pixel. The LAWS TEM feature differentiated normal and abnormal images by 12%.

Features from normal and abnormal chest X-ray images are also investigated based on the gray level run length. The normalized mean and standard deviation values of normal and abnormal images are shown in Table 3.2. The mean and standard deviation of GLRL features are able to distinguish normal and abnormal images. Features with significant differences in the mean of normal and abnormal images are highlighted. HGRE is found to be lower in abnormal subjects than normal ones. This may be due to non- uniformity in pixel intensity, which in turn leads to short runs. Short run and low gray value are high in normal subjects. This may be due to low intensity values and the homogeneous nature of the image. Runlength non-uniformity is less for normal images, which may be due to uniform distribution of the runs throughout the images. Among the GLRL features, SRHGE could differentiate normal and abnormal images by 28%.

TABLE 3.2

Normalized mean and standard deviation of GLRL features

Features	Mean ± Std dev	
	Normal Images	Abnormal Images
SRE	0.45 ± 0.23	0.45 ± 0.31
LRE	0.53 ± 030	0.42 ± 0.25
GLN	0.32 ± 0.27	0.40 ± 0.31
RLN	$\mathbf{0.31 \pm 0.27}$	$\mathbf{0.48 \pm 0.28}$
RP	0.40 ± 0.28	0.39 ± 0.31
LGRE	0.57 ± 0.24	0.43 ± 0.23
HGRE	$\mathbf{0.54 \pm 0.23}$	$\mathbf{0.39 \pm 0.34}$
SRLGE	$\mathbf{0.35 \pm 0.27}$	$\mathbf{0.52 \pm 0.32}$
SRHGE	$\mathbf{0.54 \pm 0.28}$	$\mathbf{0.26 \pm 0.36}$
LRLGE	$\mathbf{0.53 \pm 0.29}$	$\mathbf{0.39 \pm 0.26}$
LRHGE	$\mathbf{0.31 \pm 0.25}$	$\mathbf{0.44 \pm 0.31}$

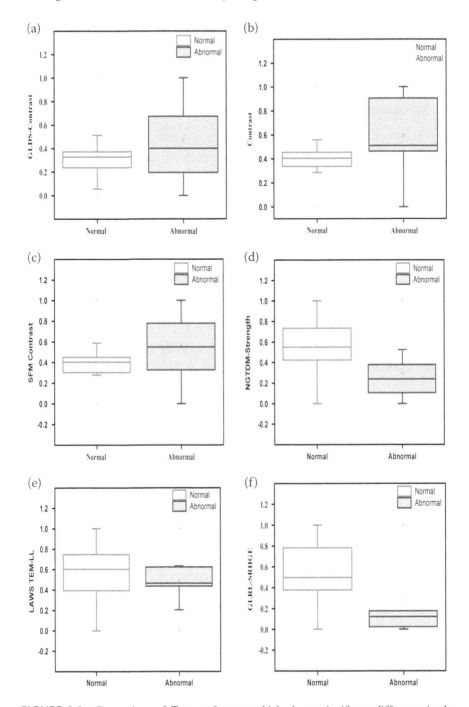

FIGURE 3.8 Comparison of Texture features which shows significant difference in the normal and abnormal features: (a) GLDS-Contrast (b) GLCM-Entropy (c) SFM Contrast (d) NGDM Strength (e) LAWS TEM-LL and (f) GLRL-SRHGE.

Chest X-rays, which are efficient in depicting visual characteristics, are analyzed using Texture features. The features which show significant difference among the normal and abnormal images are depicted using the box plot, as shown in Figure 3.8.

Figure 3.8 (a,b & c) show the high range of contrast in abnormal images. This may be due to the existence of pathology in the chest X-ray. The NGTDM feature strength extracted using neighborhood gray tone matrix differentiated normal and abnormal images. The feature extracted using LAWS mask in Figure 3.8(e) shows less difference between normal and abnormal features. Among all the features, as shown in Figure 3.8(f), the GLRL feature SRHGE has a high value in a normal, compared with an abnormal, image. The short run depicts non- uniformity in the image. Since the pixels in the normal images are uniform and smooth, the normal image is of high range.

3.4   CONCLUSION

COVID-19, the novel coronavirus disease, is a worldwide pandemic. Early diagnosis is essential to increase the survival rate. In this work, statistical texture features are extracted from normal and abnormal chest X-ray images. Extracted features are investigated to aid clinical decisions. Various texture features, such as first-order based, GLCM, NGTDM, GLDS, SFM and GLRL features, are extracted and investigated. The first-order feature Contrast differentiates normal and abnormal features by 20%. The GLDS feature obtained from gray level differences does not show prominent differences in normal and abnormal features. Entropy, which depicts the information content, is extracted from the co-occurrence matrix and found to be prominent among normal and abnormal features. The higher order NGTDM feature, based on the neighborhood gray tone difference is effective in differentiating normal and abnormal features. Among NGTDM features, Strength demarcates normal and abnormal features by 27%. Coarseness is the statistical feature extracted from the matrix; it differentiates pathological features by 20%. Texture energy extracted by LAWS mask differentiates normal and abnormal features by 12%. The feature extracted from gray level run length is also investigated in this work. SRHGE was efficient in discriminating normal and abnormal images by 28%. Coarseness, Contrast, Entropy, Strength and run-length-based features are efficient in distinguishing between normal and abnormal images. Hence, statistical texture features also play significant roles in classifying normal and abnormal images. These should be considered for screening and diagnostic purposes.

REFERENCES

Basu, S., & Mitra, S. (2020). Deep Learning for Screening COVID-19 using chest X-ray Images. *arXiv preprint arXiv:2004.10507.*

Cozzi, A., Schiaffino, S., Arpaia, F., Della Pepa, G., Tritella, S., Bertolotti, P. & Paskeh, B. B. (2020). chest X-ray in the COVID-19 pandemic: Radiologists' real-world reader performance. *European Journal of Radiology, 132*, 109272.

Dansana, D., Kumar, R., Bhattacharjee, A., Hemanth, D. J., Gupta, D., Khanna, A., & Castillo, O. (2020). Early diagnosis of COVID-19-affected patients based on X-ray and computed tomography images using deep learning algorithm. *Soft Computing*, 1–9.

Dasarathy, B. V., & Holder, E. B. (1991). Image characterizations based on joint gray level—run length distributions. *Pattern Recognition Letters*, *12*(8), 497–502.

Galloway, M. M., & Mm, G. (1975). Texture analysis using gray level run lengths.

Hamimi, A. (2016). MERS-CoV: Middle East respiratory syndrome corona virus: Can radiology be of help? Initial single center experience. *The Egyptian Journal of Radiology and Nuclear Medicine*, *47*(1), 95–106.

Han, F., Zhang, G., Wang, H., Song, B., Lu, H., Zhao, D., … & Liang, Z. (2013, October). A texture feature analysis for diagnosis of pulmonary nodules using LIDC-IDRI database. In *2013 IEEE International Conference on Medical Imaging Physics and Engineering* (pp. 14–18). IEEE.

Iqbal, H. M., Romero-Castillo, K. D., Bilal, M., & Parra-Saldivar, R. (2020). The emergence of novel-coronavirus and its replication cycle: an overview. *J Pure Appl Microbiol*, *14*(1), 13–16.

Kanne, J. P., Little, B. P., Chung, J. H., Elicker, B. M., & Ketai, L. H. (2020). Essentials for radiologists on COVID

Kermany, D., Zhang, K., & Goldbaum, M. (2018). Labeled optical coherence tomography (OCT) and chest X-ray images for classification. *Mendeley Data*, 2.

Kim, H. W., Capaccione, K. M., Li, G., Luk, L., Widemon, R. S., Rahman, O., … & Dumeer, S. (2020). The role of initial chest X-ray in triaging patients with suspected COVID-19 during the pandemic. *Emergency Radiology*, *27*(6), 617–621,

Li J., Xu Z., Zhang Y. (2018) *Diagnosing chest X-ray diseases with deep learning* (pp. 1–6). Stanford University.

Loizou, C. P., Petroudi, S., Seimenis, I., Pantziaris, M., & Pattichis, C. S. (2015). Quantitative texture analysis of brain white matter lesions derived from T2-weighted MR images in MS patients with clinically isolated syndrome. *Journal of Neuroradiology*, *42*(2), 99–114.

Murphy, K., Smits, H., Knoops, A. J., Korst, M. B., Samson, T., Scholten, E. T., … & Melendez, J. (2020). COVID-19 on the chest radiograph: A multi-reader evaluation of an AI system. *Radiology*, *296*(3), E166–E172.

Parry, A. H., & Wani, A. H. (2020). Pulmonary embolism in coronavirus disease-19 (COVID-19) and use of compression ultrasonography in its optimal management. *Thrombosis Research*, *192*, 36.

Rachidi, M., Chappard, C., Marchadier, A., Gadois, C., Lespessailles, E., & Benhamou, C. L. (2008, May). Application of Laws' masks to bone texture analysis: An innovative image analysis tool in osteoporosis. In *2008 5th IEEE International Symposium on Biomedical Imaging: From Nano to Macro* (pp. 1191–1194). IEEE.

Salehi, S., Abedi, A., Balakrishnan, S., &Gholamrezanezhad, A. (2020). Coronavirus disease 2019 (COVID-19): a systematic review of imaging findings in 919 patients. *American Journal of Roentgenology*, *215*(1), 87–93.

Siddiqui, M. K., Morales-Menendez, R., Gupta, P. K., Iqbal, H. M., Hussain, F., Khatoon, K., & Ahmad, S. (2020). Correlation between temperature and COVID-19 (suspected, confirmed and death) cases based on machine learning analysis. *Journal ofPure and Applied Microbiology*, *14*(suppl 1), 1017–1024.

Silva, P., Luz, E., Silva, G., Moreira, G., Silva, R., Lucio, D., & Menotti, D. (2020). COVID-19 detection in CT images with deep learning: A voting-based scheme and cross-datasets analysis. *Informatics in Medicine Unlocked*, *20*, 100427.

Srinivasan, G. N., & Shobha, G. (2008, December). Statistical texture analysis. *Proceedings of World Academy of Science, Engineering and Technology*, *36*, 1264–1269.

Sun, Z., Zhang, N., Li, Y., & Xu, X. (2020). A systematic review of chest imaging findings in COVID-19. *Quantitative Imaging in Medicine and Surgery, 10*(5), 1058.

Su, S., Wong, G., Shi, W., Liu, J., Lai, A. C., Zhou, J., Liu, W., Bi, Y., & Gao, G. F. (2016). Epidemiology, genetic recombination, and pathogenesis of coronaviruses. *Trends in Microbiology, 24*(6), 490–502.

Wang, W., Xu, Y., Gao, R., Lu, R., Han, K., Wu, G., & Tan, W. (2020). Detection of SARS

World health organization: https://www.who.int/new-room/g-a-detail/q-a-corronaviruses# :/text=symptoms. Accessed 10 Apr 2020.

Xie, X., Li, X., Wan, S., & Gong, Y. (2006). Mining x-ray images of SARS patients. In *Data Mining* (pp. 282–294). Springer, Berlin, Heidelberg.

Yang, Y., Yang, M., Shen, C., Wang, F., Yuan, J., Li, J., … & Peng, L. (2020). Laboratory diagnosis and monitoring the viral shedding of 2019. *The Innovation, 1*(3), 100061.

Zhu, N., Zhang, D., Wang, W., Li, X., Yang, B., Song, J., & Niu, P. (2020). A novel coronavirus from patients with pneumonia in China, 2019. *New England Journal of Medicine, 328*(8), 727–733.

4 Efficient Diagnosis using Chest CT in COVID-19: A Review

J. Sivakamasundari[1] *and K. Venkatesh*[2]

[1]Department of Biomedical Engineering, Jerusalem College of Engineering, Chennai, India
[2]Kovai Medical Center and Hospital, Coimbatore, India

4.1 INTRODUCTION

On 11 March 2020, the World Health Organisation (WHO) declared COVID-19 a pandemic. It is an infectious disease which affects human lungs and causes severe pneumonia (World 2020). The first case was reported in Wuhan, China during December 2019. It is still spreading worldwide primarily by human transmission through respiratory droplets produced when coughing and sneezing. Globally, more than 43.56 million people have been infected; among those, there were 1.16 million deaths as of October 2020 (Wuhan 2020).

COVID-19 infection shows symptoms such as fever, cough, fatigue, headache, haemoptysis, diarrhoea, shortness of breath, and odour and taste disturbances. People with mild clinical symptoms may not require hospitalization, but clinical signs such as fever, cough and difficulty in breathing may develop into lower-respiratory-tract disease. 97.5% of patients developed symptoms within 12 days of exposure but, for old and weak patients, particularly with comorbidities, this disease caused severe lung infections within a few days and led to death (Davide et al. 2020). This infection initiates clusters of respiratory complications, such as severe pneumonia, acute respiratory distress syndrome (ARDS), secondary to massive alveolar injury, acute cerebrovascular injury, renal and liver failure, any of which may cause death (Huang et al. 2020).

Common measures to prevent the disease include frequent hand washing and maintaining distance from other people. Avoiding touching the face repeatedly and using masks are also recommended for those suspected of having this virus. Currently, development of specific antiviral treatments or vaccines are in the testing phase. Hence, rapid and accurate identification methods, treatment of symptoms and supportive hospital care are important issues in the diagnosis and control of COVID-19 (Neelesh et al. 2020). Recent studies address the importance of imaging techniques using radiology. Chest CT and X-ray images contain significant COVID-19 findings, even for patients who receive false negative RT-PCR test results. Application of advanced detection algorithms along with radiological image findings allow physicians to make the best decisions in detecting this disease (Tulin et al. 2020). The sensitivity of chest X-rays for initial symptoms of SARS-CoV-2 pneumonia is less than (57%). It becomes higher more than five days from the day of exposure and slightly higher in elderly patients than younger ones (Davide et al. 2020). Chest CT imaging plays a vital role in early diagnosis of COVID-19; its sensitivity is reported as 98% (Xie et al. 2020).

The progression of this disease is having severe impact on all over the world. Chest CT is the most valuable imaging tool for the clinical diagnosis of early stage COVID19 pneumonia when disease symptoms are nonspecific. Several investigations on radiological images have been carried out by researchers for early detection of this infection (Kong and Agarwal 2020). Various abnormal disease findings in lungs, such as right or left infrahilar airspace opacities and the presence of single nodular opacity or irregular opacities in both lungs are observed in a COVID-19 infected patient (Pan et al. 2020, Xiong et al. 2020).

Radiographic findings, such as ground glass opacities (GGO) or mixed GGO, consolidation, and vascular dilation in lesions, are also observed in COVID-19 patients (Zhao et al. 2020). Abnormal lesions present in the peripheral and posterior lung fields are called mixed ground glass opacities and consolidation or pure ground-glass opacities, which are considered COVID-19 findings (Yoon et al. 2020). Other common chest CT image features of COVID-19 patients are GGO, consolidation, interlobular septal thickening and air bronchogram signs, with or without vascular expansion (Li and Xia 2020). This chapter describes the clinical significance of chest CT imaging used as a diagnostic aid for COVID-19-affected high-risk patients.

4.2   CLINICAL EVALUATIONS

Several screening methods are followed in the detection of SARS-Cov-2. RT-PCR test is a standard diagnostic procedure recommended for all infected patients involving a sample of nasopharyngeal or oropharyngeal swab. This method has limitations, including accessibility and availability (Xie et al. 2020). Sometimes the sensitivity of RT-PCR becomes as low as 60%–70%, and can show negative results. In that case, symptoms of pneumonia are detected by investigating radiological images (Kanne et al. 2020). Other methods, such as serological tests based on immunoglobulin M (IgM)/IgG antibody detection, which includes ELISA tests and rapid chromatographic tests, are also adopted in COVID-19 detection. Advantages of these tests are rapid results, high sensitivity (~89%) and specificity (~93%), easy accessibility and fast screening for COVID-19 infections (Neelesh et al. 2020).

A study was carried out in Singapore for 70 patients. They were subjected to the PCR test for SARS-CoV-2. In the first round of testing, 62 out of 70 patients were diagnosed as COVID-19 positive. In the second round of testing, 24 hours after the first test, five more patients were diagnosed as positive whose initial results were negative. In the third round of testing, results of the three remaining patients became positive (Lee et al. 2020). This study shows that infected patients with comorbidities should not wait for repeated testing. This is not safe for high-risk patients.

4.3   IMAGE INTERPRETATIONS

The chest x-ray is easily available and rapidly interpretable compared to other imaging modalities. CXR usually shows bilateral infiltrates, but sometimes shows normal in the early stages of the disease. CXR images are convenient for investigation and useful in diagnosing other coronaviruses such as severe acute respiratory syndrome (SARS) and Middle East respiratory syndrome (MERS) (Franks et al. 2003, Kaw et al. 2003, Tsou et al. 2004, Ahmed et al. 2018). In SARS-CoV-2 pneumonia, the sensitivity of CXR is 57%. For asymptomatic patients, sensitivity and specificity are comparatively low (Davide et al. 2020). Sensitivity of CXR increases with time, and repeated CXR imaging may provide the clear indications of SARS-CoV-2 infection shows characteristic CXR signs, such as patchy and confluent, bandlike GGO or consolidation in aperipheral and distribution from middle-to-lower lung zone. It exhibits efficient diagnosis when its findings are correlated with clinical RT-PCR test results (Lorente 2020).

Research was conducted on COVID-19 patients based on CXR imaging. Figure 4.1 (a-c) shows the CXR images of a 63-year-old female suffering from dyspnea and fever, a 41-year-old female affected by fever and cough, and a 41-year-old male with dyspnea and chest pain respectively (Smith et al. 2020). The arrows which are shown in Figure 4.1(a) evidently proves the findings such as bilateral – patchy and confluent, bandlike ground glass and consolidative opacity in peripheral and middle-to-lower lung zone.

Figure 4.1(b) illustrates the characteristics of CXR findings called bilateral-patchy and confluent, band like ground glass and consolidative opacity in a peripheral, mid-to-lower lung zone distribution pointed by arrows. Figure 4.1(c) shows the patchy GGO which are limited to the peripheral portions of mid-lung zones, shown by arrows. From images (a-c) it is evident that, though chest radiographs are low in sensitivity, they may be indicated for COVID-19 patients. They can be used along with positive RT-PCR test results, but they are not a substitute for RT-PCR test or chest CT.

(a)   (b)   (c)

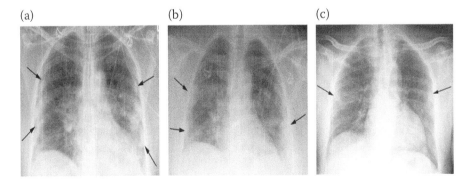

FIGURE 4.1   Characteristic CXR images. (a) and (b) Bilateral patchy and confluent, bandlike ground glass and consolidative opacity in a peripheral, mid-to-lower lung zone distribution pointed by arrows, (c) Patchy ground glass opacities are limited to the peripheral portions of the mid lung zones pointed by arrows (Smith et al., 2020).

Another study was carried out on a 50-year-old patient infected by COVID-19 pneumonia. CXR images taken at days one, four, five and seven are shown in Figure 4.2(a-d). From Figure 4.2(a) it is observed that the X-ray taken on day one shows clear lungs with no significant findings of COVID-19 infection. Figure 4.2(b), taken on the fourth day of infection, exhibits patchy and abnormal bilateral alveolar consolidations with peripheral distribution. Figure 4.2(c) shows a severely abnormal condition with consolidation in the left upper lobe on the fifth day. Figure 4.2(d) illustrates the severely abnormal condition with distinctive

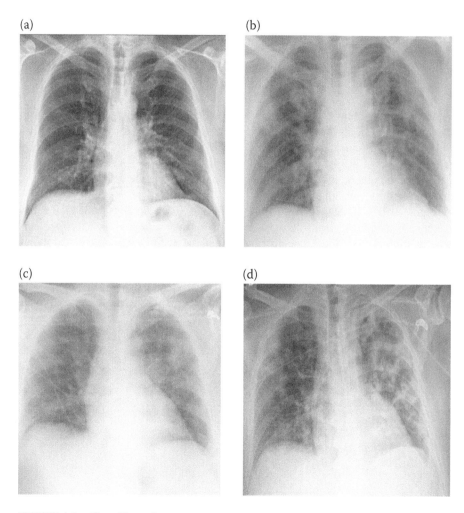

FIGURE 4.2   Chest X-ray images taken at days 1, 4, 5 and 7 respectively for a 50 year old COVID-19 patient with pneumonia. (a) Clear lungs with no significant findings on day 1, (b) Patchy, ill-defined bilateral alveolar consolidations, with a peripheral distribution on day 4, (c) Degenerative condition with consolidation in the left upper lobe on day 5 and (d) Degenerative state with typical findings of ARDS on day 7 (Edgar Lorente 2020).

findings of acute respiratory distress syndrome (ARDS) infection on the seventh day (Lorente 2020).

Figure 4.1 and 4.2 suggest that radiographic images could present fast, cost-effective diagnoses for COVID-19-infected patients, but not in the early stages. CXR does not show findings when the virus has spread to the upper respiratory area, such as nose and throat. The effectiveness of this imaging is higher when the infection is in advanced stage, meaning it is in mid-to-lower lung zone or lower respiratory tract, called pneumonia. Hence it may not be helpful for elderly and high-risk patients with one or more comorbidities.

During the initial stages of the pandemic, clinical laboratories had insufficient test kits and more false negative results were provided. Therefore, doctors were advised to take decisions based on laboratory results combined with chest CT results for early detection (Kong and Agarwal 2020, Li and Xia 2020, Bernheim et al. 2020, Lee et al. 2020, Long et al. 2020, Shi et al. 2020, Zhao et al. 2020). CT scan shows fine findings (like severity of lung infiltration) more accurate which can be missed in X-Ray. Particularly, CT scan imaging provides unambiguous findings when investigating the severity of lung infiltration. Some limitations of CT scans are greater time requirements, less availability of CT scanners, and implementation of social distancing and standard sanitizing methods after the scan (Levine and Caputo 2020). Chest CT images give evidence of many significant features of disease severity in COVID-19 patients when taken in different time periods (Ye et al. 2020).

Several studies have interpreted chest CT images of patients with COVID-19 symptoms and other lung complications and abnormalities, depending on stage and severity of the disease (Kwee 2020). Various chest CTs show abnormal conditions related to COVID-19 pneumonia in confirmed cases, including GGOs, consolidation, mixed GGO and consolidation, traction bronchiectasis, thickening of bronchial wall, reticulation, and subpleural bands. Multi-plane views such as transverse, sagittal, and coronal, are helpful for decision making when nucleic acid tests results are negative (Ajlan et al. 2014).

CT image abnormalities related to lung infections are explained in various research papers. Ground glass opacity means, increased lung density with no obscuration of underlying lung markings. Consolidation means increased lung density due to abnormal lung markings. Perilobular opacities are polygonal or curvilinear bands in the adjoining secondary pulmonary lobule area. Interlobular or intralobular irregular septal thickening is called reticulation. Thin linear opacities like subpleural bands are situated in peripheral and parallel to the pleura. Irregular or dilated airways in areas of fibrosis are termed traction bronchiectasis (Thomas and Robert 2020).

Chest CT scanning for COVID-19-associated pneumonia usually shows GGO with consolidation and other abnormalities, which are generally bilateral and spread around the lower lobes of lungs. Accumulation of fluids between the chest wall and the lungs causes an infection, called pleural effusion, and formation of scar tissues, called pleural thickening. These are also reported in recent research (Davide et al. 2020).

Figure 4.3 shows radiological images of a 59-year-old COVID-19-infected woman. Figure 4.3(a) shows the chest X-ray with findings of right infrahilar airspace opacities; Figure 4.3(b-e) are lung CT images. Figure 4.3(b) axial and (c) sagittal images exhibit GGOs in the peripherallower right lobe of lungs. Figure 4.3(d) axial and (e) sagittal chest CT images, taken two days later, show improvement in the GGOs, with extended sub-pleural curvilinear lines, indicated by arrows (Kong and Agarwal 2020).

Chest CT images taken from a COVID-19 patient are shown in Figure 4.4. A small single nodular GGO in the left upper lobe is shown in Figure 4.4(a) and its progression in three days to multifocal nodularis is clearly shown in Figure 4.4(b). Peripheral GGO involving both upper lobes is unambiguously exhibited in Figure 4.4(c). Another follow-up CT taken five days from the presentation is illustrated in Figure 4.4(d); it shows a new tiny cavity. Figure 4.4(e) points up an increase in abnormality of consolidation with GGOs and septal thickening (Kong and Agarwal 2020).

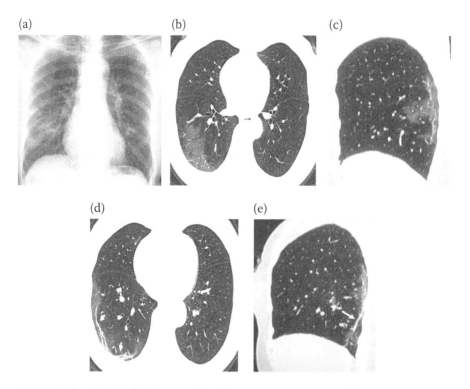

FIGURE 4.3   Radiological images of a 59-year-old woman with COVID-19 infection.
(a) Chest X-ray of right infrahilar airspace opacities, (b) axial, (c) sagittal view of lung CT images taken from peripherallower right lobe GGOs, (d) axial, (e) lung CT in sagittal view taken after 2 days shows more GGOs, with extended sub-pleural curvilinear lines given in arrows (Kong and Agarwal 2020).

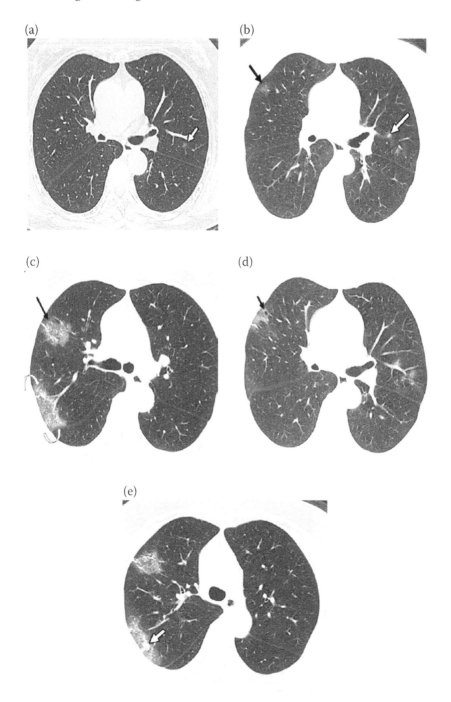

FIGURE 4.4 Chest CT taken from a COVID patient. (a) Multifocal nodular after three days progression, (b) and (c) Peripheral GGOs involving both upper lobes, (d) CT image taken five days from infection showing new tiny cavity and (e) increased consolidation mixed with GGOs and crazy-paving pattern (Kong and Agarwal 2020).

In the pandemic situation, a study was conducted on patients suffering with cough and dizziness without fever. Their initial RT-PCR results showed weakly positive on the first swab test. Chest CT scan and a second swab test were conducted the next day. The swab test was negative, but chest CT examination confirmed viral pneumonia. The third swab test was taken two days later and was positive for COVID-19. This study suggests that a typical CT finding helps in early screening of lung complications (Xie et al. 2020).

Figure 4.5 shows abnormalities observed from a chest CT scan taken from a COVID-19-confirmed patient on different days of illness; the day initial symptoms are seen is day 0. Figure 4.5(a) shows abnormalities such as ground-glass with intralobular septal thickening (also known as a crazy-paving pattern) present in lower right lobe of the lung from images taken on day three of the illness. Opacity is marked by a white arrow. A scan taken on the seventh day of infection shows intralobular septal thickening in addition to increased patchy GGO. This was newly

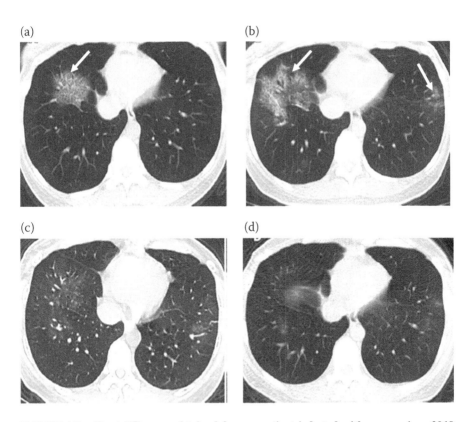

FIGURE 4.5 Chest CT scans obtained from a patient infected with coronavirus 2019 pneumonia. (a) Third day of illness illustrates GGO with intralobular septal thickening in lower right lobe, (b) Seventh day image shows intralobular septal thickening combined on GGOand increased patchy GGO in lower left lobe, (c) 12th day image evediently shows reduced abnormalities with pure GGO in both lower lobes on and (d) 17th day scan clearly shows pure GGO in both lower lobes (Wang et al. 2020).

(a)   (b)   (c)

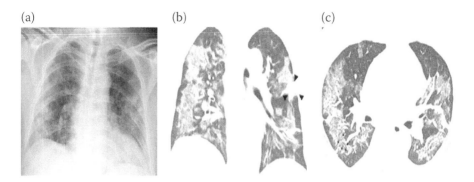

FIGURE 4.6   Chest images show COVID-19 infection. (a) Chest X-ray, (b) Coronal and axial chest CT images with confluent mixed ground-glass opacities, (c) Axial CT image which shows evidence of confluent lesions (Yoon et al. 2020).

developed in the lower left lobe, marked in white arrows in Figure 4.5(b). A scan taken on the 12th day shows reduction in abnormalities and absence of GGOs in both lower lobes, as shown in Figure 4.5(c). In the scan taken on the 17th day, pure GGOs are observed on both lobes in lower region as show in Figure 4.5(d). On the 20th day of illness, the patient was discharged (Wang et al. 2020).

Figure 4.6 presents chest X-ray and CT images consistent with COVID-19 pneumonia findings. Figure 4.6(a) illustrates the anteroposterior chest X-ray with multifocal patchy peripheral consolidations in the upper side of the right lung area. Figure 4.6(b) and (c) represent the coronal and axial chest CT images with confluent mixed GGOs and consolidative lesions in peripheral bilateral lungs. Discrete patchy consolidations specified by arrows are shown in the upper left lobe of the lung. Figure 4.6(c) represents the axial CT image which shows evidence of confluent lesions, mainly distributed in the peripheral lung along bronchovascular bundles. It also shows lesions present in the juxtapleural area and those touching pleura. Lesions are present in the superior segment of the lower right lobe, which contains multiple air-bronchograms and is slightly distorted (Yoon et al. 2020).

COVID-19 findings in chest X-ray and CT scan images of a patient are shown in Figure 4.7(a-c). The baseline anteroposterior chest radiograph with patchy GGOs appear on upper and lower zones of the right lung, as shown in Figure 4.7(a). It also shows patchy consolidation in middle to lower zones of left lung. More calcified granulomas are observed in the upper left lung zone. Figure 4.7(b) is the baseline axial chest CT image which shows confluent pure GGOs spread over on both lungs. Figure 4.7(c) is the coronal chest CT image, which shows confluent and patchy GGOs about the pleura and fissures in the peripheral lung. Some small calcified granulomas are also seen in the upper left lobe (Yoon et al. 2020). Figure 4.7 shows that chest CT findings are clearer than CXR.

Figure 4.8(a) represents the anteroposterior CXR of a patient affected by COVID-19 pneumonia. From (a) it is observed that a nodular lesion with consolidation is present in lower left lung area. The chest CT image (b), evidently exhibits a 2.3 cm nodular lesion. It was imaged on the same day the X-ray was

(a)   (b)   (c)

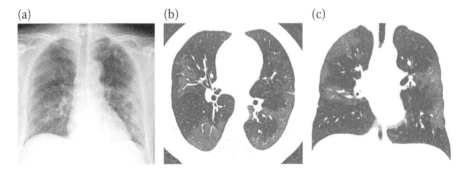

FIGURE 4.7   Representative chest X-ray and CT images. (a) Chest X-ray represents patchy ground-glass opacities in lower lung and patchy consolidation in left-mid-lower zone, (b) Baseline axial chest CT image illustrates confluent pure ground-glass opacities in peripheral lung (c) Baseline coronal chest CT image exhibits patchy ground-glass opacities and granulomas in upper left lobe (Yoon et al. 2020).

taken (Yoon et al. 2020). This study also proves that the chest CT findings of COVID-19 are more significant and instantly recognizable than CXR.

Chest X-ray images and Chest CT scan images are compared in Figures 4.6, 4.7 and 4.8 based on their significance and clarity in COVID-19 findings. From all the representative chest CT images it is observed that COVID-19 findings and the progression of the illness are shown more clearly than in chest X-ray images. In chest CT, COVID-19 pneumonia is observed as pure GGO to mixed GGO and lesions are consolidative in the bilateral peripheral posterior lungs. The shape of the lesions proves their abnormality and explicitly indicates the distribution of patchy

(a)   (b)

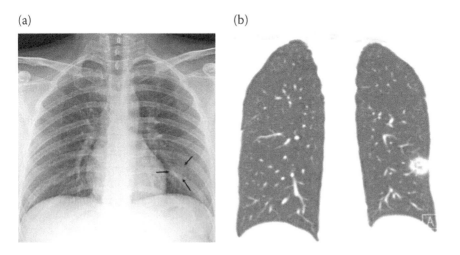

FIGURE 4.8   Findings of chest X-ray and chest CT images of a COVID-19 person. (a) X-ray represents single nodular lesion and (b) CT scan image represents single nodular lesion in lungs (Yoon et al. 2020).

nodular lesions along bronchovascular bundles over the pleura. In chest X-ray images, pulmonary lesions are ambiguous and difficult to investigate.

4.4 CONCLUSION

Chest X-ray and computed tomography image findings are significant in the detection of lung complications. Though the sensitivity of chest X-ray is 57% for COVID-19 detection, it is not recommended for patients with early stage of COVID-19 infections. Chest CT images demonstrate almost all abnormalities, including mild lesions. It is advised to diagnose COVID-19 in its early stages. Routine chest X-ray findings are widely used in diagnosis of respiratory symptoms such as cough, dyspnea, pneumonia and complications like pleural effusion or abscess formation. Chest CT findings are helpful to detect abnormalities not detectable with chest radiograph, due to higher sensitivity (98%). Hence, clinicians and radiologists must get adequate knowledge about chest CT findings related to COVID-19 infection, existing degree of severity, combined clinical symptoms and laboratory tests. This could facilitate the comprehensive prevention, efficient diagnosis, isolation and treatment of COVID-19 pneumonia.

REFERENCES

Ahmed A. E., Jahdali H. A., Alshukairi A. N., Alaqeel M., Siddiq S. S., Alsaab H., Sakr E. A., Alyahya H. A., Alandonisi M. M., Subedar A. T., Aloudah N. M., Baharoon S., Alsalamah M. A., Johani S. A. and Alghamdi M. G. 2018. Early identification of pneumonia patients at increased risk of Middle East respiratory syndrome coronavirus infection in Saudi Arabia. *International Journal of Infectious Diseases* 70:51–56, https://doi.org/10.1016/j.ijid.2018.03.005.

Ajlan A. M., Ahyad R. A., Jamjoom L. G., Alharthy A. and Madani T. A. 2014. Middle East respiratory syndrome coronavirus (MERS-CoV) infection: chest CT findings. *American Journal of Roentgenology* 203(4):782–787.

Bernheim A., Mei X., Huang M., Yang Y., Fayad Z. A., Zhang N., Diao K., Lin B., Zhu X., Li K., Li S., Shan H., Jacobi A. and Chung M. 2020. Chest CT findings in coronavirus disease-19 (COVID-19): relationship to duration of infection. *Radiology* 295:685–691. https://doi.org/10.1148/radiol.2020200463.

Davide I., Anna P., Cesare M., Carlo C., Ilaria M., Teresa G., Davide G., Ilaria B., Maria R., Cammillo T. F., Rocco C. and Sandro S. 2020. Diagnostic impact of bedside chest X-ray features of 2019 novel coronavirus in the routine admission at the emergency department: case series from Lombardy region. *European Journal of Radiology*, 129:1–6.

Franks T. J., Chong P. Y., Chui P., Galvin J. R., Lourens R. M., Reid A. H., Selbs E., McEvoy C. P., Hayden C. D., Fukuoka J., Taubenberger J. K. and Travis W. D. 2003. Lung pathology of severe acute respiratory syndrome (SARS): a study of 8 autopsy cases from Singapore. *Human Pathology*, 34:743–748, https://doi.org/10.1016/s0046-8177(03)00367-8.

Huang C., Wang Y., Li X., Ren L., Zhao J., Hu Y., Zhang L., Fan G., Xu J., Gu X., Cheng Z., Yu T., Xia J., Wei Y., Wu W., Xie X., Yin W., Li H., Liu M., Xiao Y., Gao H., Guo L., Xie J., Wang G., Jiang R., Gao Z., Jin Q., Wang J. and Cao B. 2020. *Clinical features of patients infected with 2019 novel coronavirus in Wuhan, China.* Lancet (London, England).

Kanne J. P., Little B. P., Chung J. H., Elicker B. M. and Ketai L. H. 2020. Essentials for radiologists on COVID-19: an update—radiology scientific expert panel. *Radiology* 296:E113–E114. https://doi.org/10.1148/radiol.2020200527.

Kaw G. J., Tan D. Y., Leo Y. S., Tsou I. Y., Wansaicheong G. and Chee T. S. 2003. Chest radiographic findings of a case of severe acute respiratory syndrome (SARS) in Singapore. *Singapore Medical Journal* 44(4):201–204.

Kong W. and Agarwal P. P. 2020. Chest imaging appearance of COVID-19 infection. *Radiology: Cardiothoracic Imaging* 2(1).

Kwee T. C. and Kwee R. M. 2020. Chest CT in COVID-19: what the radiologist needs to know. *RadioGraphics* 40:1846–1865.

Kwee T. C., and Kwee R. M. 2020. Chest CT in COVID-19: What the radiologist needs to know.*RadioGraphics*40(7): 1848–1865.

Lee T. H., Lin R. J., Lin R. T. P., Barkham T., Rao P., Leo Y. S., Lye D. C. and Young B. 2020. Testing for SARS-CoV-2: can we stop at two? *Clinical Infectious Diseases* 71(16):2246–2248. https://doi.org/10.1093/cid/ciaa459.

Lee E. Y., Ng M. Y. and Khong P. L. 2020. COVID-19 pneumonia: what has CT taught us?. *Lancet Infectious Diseases* 20(4):384–385.

Levine R. and Caputo N. 2020. CT scan of a COVID-positive patient. *Journal of the American College of Emergency Physician Open* 1(2):143–147.

Li L., Qin L., Xu Z., Yin Y., Wang X., Kong B., Bai J., Lu Y., Fang Z., Song Q., Cao K., Liu D., Wang G., Xu Q., Fang X., Zhang S., Xia J., Xia J. 2020. Using artificial intelligence to detect COVID-19 and community-acquired pneumonia based on pulmonary CT: evaluation of the diagnostic accuracy. *Radiology* 296(2): E65–E7.

Li Y. and Xia L. 2020. Coronavirus disease 2019 (COVID-19): role of chest CT in diagnosis and management. *American Journal of Roentgenology* 214(6): 1280–1286.

Long C., Xu H., Shen Q., Zhang X., Fan B., Wang C., Zeng B. Li Z., Li X. and Li H. 2020. Diagnosis of the Coronavirus disease (COVID-19): rRT-PCR or CT?. *European Journal of Radiology* 126:108961.

Lorente E., COVID-19 pneumonia - evolution over a week. https://radiopaedia.org/cases/COVID-19-pneumonia-evolution-over-a-week-1?lang¼us.

Neelesh J., Animesh C., Jayesh S., Venkata K., Divyendu D. and Richa T. 2020. A review of novel coronavirus infection (*Coronavirus Disease*-19) 5(1):22–26.

Pan Y., Guan H., Zhou S., Wang Y., Li Q., Zhu T., Hu Q. and Xia L. 2020. Initial CT findings and temporal changes in patients with the novel coronavirus pneumonia (SARS-CoV-2): a study of 63 patients in Wuhan, China.*European Journal of Radiology*, 30(6), 3306–3309, https://doi.org/10.1007/s00330-020-06731-x.

Shi H., Han X., Jiang N., Cao Y., Alwalid O., Gu J., Fan Y. and Zheng C. 2020. Radiological findings from 81 patients with COVID-19 pneumonia in Wuhan, China: a descriptive study. *Lancet Infectious Diseases* 24(4):425–434.

Singh D., Vijay Kumar, V. and Kaur M. 2020. Classification of COVID-19 patients from chest CT images using multi-objective differential evolution–based convolutional neural networks. *European Journal of Clinical Microbiology & Infectious Diseases*, 39(7), 1379–1389.

Smith D. L., Grenierm J. P., Batte C. and Spieler B. 2020. A characteristic chest radiographic pattern in the setting of COVID-19 pandemic. *Radiology: Cardiothoracic Imaging* 2(5): e200280 DOI: 10.1148/ryct.2020200280.

Tsou I. Y., Loh L. E., Kaw G. J., Chan I. and Chee T. S. 2004. Severe acute respiratory syndrome (SARS) in a paediatric cluster in Singapore. *Pediatric Radiology* 34(1):43–46. https://doi.org/10.1007/s00247-003-1042-2.

Tulin O., Muhammed T., Eylul A. Y., Ulas B. B., Ozal Y. and Rajendra A. 2020. Automated detection of COVID-19 cases using deep neural networks with X-ray images. *Computers in Biology and Medicine*, 121, 4–11.

Wang Y., Dong C., Hu Y., Li C., Ren Q., Zhang X., Shi H. and Zhou M. 2020. Temporal changes of CT findings in 90 patients with COVID-19 pneumonia: a longitudinal study. *Radiology* 296:E55–E64.

World Health Organization website. Naming the coronavirus disease (COVID-2019) and the virus that causes it. www.who.int/emergencies/diseases/novel-coronavirus2019/technical-guidance/naming-the-coronavirus-disease-(covid-2019)andthe-virus-that-causes-it. Published 2020. Accessed February26, 2020

Wuhan Coronavirus (2019-nCoV) Global cases (by Johns Hopkins CSSE). *Case Dashboard.* (Accessed 27 October 2020).

Xie X., Zhong Z., Zhou W., Zheng C., Wang F. and Liu J. 2020. Chest CT for typical 2019-nCoV pneumonia: relationship to negative RTPCR testing. *Radiology.* https://doi.org/10.1148/radiol.2020200343.

Xiong Y., Sun D., Liu Y., Fan Y., Zhao L., Li X. and Zhu W. 2020. Clinical and highresolution CT features of the COVID-19 infection: comparison of the initial and follow-up changes. *Investigative Radiology* https://doi.org/10.1007/s00330-020-06731-x.

Ye Z., Zhang Y., Wang Y., Huang Z. and Song B. 2020. Chest CT manifestations of new coronavirus disease 2019 (COVID-19): a pictorial review. *European Radiology* 30:4381–4389.

Yoon S. H., Lee K. H., Kim J. Y., Lee Y. K., Ko H., Kim K. H., Park C. M. and Kim Y. H. 2020. Chest radiographic and CT findings of the 2019 novel coronavirus disease (COVID-19): analysis of nine patients treated in Korea. *Korean Journal of Radiology* 21(4):494–500. https://doi.org/10.3348/kjr.2020.0132.

Zhao W., Zhong Z., Xie X., Yu Q. and Liu J. 2020. Relation between chest CT findings and clinical conditions of coronavirus disease (COVID-19) pneumonia: a multicenter study. *American Journal of Roentgenology* 214(5):1072–1077.

5 Automatic Mask Detection and Social Distance Alerting Based on a Deep-Learning Computer Vision Algorithm

N. Vinoth[*], *A. Ganesh Ram, M. Vijayakarthick, and S. Meyyappan*

Department of Instrumentation Engineering, Madras Institute of Technology Campus, Anna University, Chennai 600044

[*]Corresponding author: vinothbalaji@rediffmail.com

5.1 INTRODUCTION

India is the second most-populated country in the world; hence, it is suffering terribly from COVID-19 (Ghosh et al., 2020). The situation worsens even after implementing lockdown and other measures taken by the Indian Government (Mehta, Jha 2020). Due to this pandemic, the Indian Economy has been tumbling like a ship into the deep sea (Gopalan, Misra 2020). Considering these scenarios, the Indian Government is phasing out lockdowns. No antiviral vaccine is yet available for COVID-19. There is a big trade-off between human lives and economic stabilization (Mahato et al., 2020).

Many sectors have been reopened in the process of lifting lockdown gradually. Within a few months schools, colleges and universities will likely reopen. During reopening, youngsters will be exposed to the outside environment, especially in their academic institutions. This may lead to an increase in cases, as the children may be liable to spread the disease. Temperature checks with non-contact thermometers (Infrared) are the major solutions around India for diagnosing. Diagnosing is done by security personnel manually; they also instruct people to wear masks(Mehta, Jha 2020). The aim of this work is to automate image capture of people who are not wearing masks, using a computer vision algorithm. It also detects whether social distance is maintained; if not, an alarm will sound as a reminder.

Mask detection is one of the key issues considered in this work. Conventionally, video is converted into a series of images. Processing of images is carried out by pre-processing techniques such as removing noise and enhancing image quality. Next, segmentation of images is done to identify the Region of Interest (ROI). The features of the images are extracted and finally, the images are classified accordingly. These methods work exceedingly well for small datasets. For huge datasets, thankfully transfer learning provides handful solution (Nieto-Rodríguez et al., 2015, Roy et al., 2020).

Image classification, speech recognition and natural language processing are the broad areas where deep-learning networks have been implemented. The deep-learning method has multiple layers between input and output, called hidden layers, which are utilized to interpret the features of input data (Lecun et al., 2015). Object detection is one form of deep learning which has evolved as giant technique for detecting objects from an image or video. Object detection is a tough task when compared to image classification, since precise localization of ROI is to be detected (Deng et al., 2009). The phenomenal development of graphics processing unit (GPU) handles a huge volume of datasets and provides efficient computing power. Evolution of various Convolutional Neural Network (CNN) models revolutionized image classification into the next stage as object detection. A few of the popular variations that have been successfully incorporated in object detection are Resnet, VGG net, Mask R-CNN and Faster R-CNN (Deng et al., 2009).

The architecture of the Convolutional Neural Network model consists of many convolution layers, pooling layers and fully-connected layers, as shown in Figure 5.1 (Huang et al., 2018). Filtering and smoothing operations are carried out in these layers of CNN. AlexNet is the basis of modern CNN, which is comprised of eight convolution layers, three pooling layers, and three fully connected layers, with Relu as the activation function. A plethora of improvisations, inspired by AlexNet, came into existence: VGGNet; GoogleNet; and ResNet. These accumulated convolution layers, pooling layers and fully connected layers (Szegedy et al., 2016).

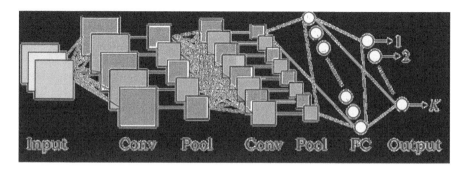

FIGURE 5.1   Typical CNN architecture.

The purpose of generic object detection is to locate and identify current objects in any single image and to labeling them with rectangular bounding boxes to signify the confidences of existence (Uijlings et al., 2013).

Generic object detection system systems can primarily be divided into two groups (see Figure 5.1). One follows the conventional pipeline for object detection, initially generating region proposals and then classifying each proposal into different categories of objects (Viola and Michael J., 2004). Another one views object identification as an issue of regression or classification; it follows a unified structure to achieve final results explicitly i.e., categories and places (Krizhevsky et al., 2017). Methods focused on the regional proposal mainly include RCNN (Ren et al., 2016) R FCN (Dai et al., 2016), FPN (Lin et al., 2017) and Mask R CNN (He et al., 2017), some of which are correlated with each other. Methods based on regression classification mainly include MultiBox (Erhan et al., 2014), AttentionNet (Yoo et al., 2015), GCNN (Najibi et al., 2016), YOLO V1 (Dai et al., 2016), SSD (Liu et al., 2016) and (Yoo et al., 2015), and YOLO V3 (Redmon, Farhadi, 2017). Using the faster RCNN bridges, the authors implemented correlations between these two pipelines.

In vast research areas it has been recognized that the Convolution Neural Network (CNN) as fastest detection method. Krizhevsky et al. (2017) implemented CNN for classification problem and won the competition of ILSVRC (ImageNet Large Scale Visual Recognition Challenge), in which he achieved in reducing the top 5 error rate to 15.3%. Previously (Krizhevsky et al., 2012) has proposed Region Convolutional Neural Network (RCNN) through fucsioned the RPN (Region Proposal Network) and CNN methods, which were tested on Pascal VOC 2007, which yielded the mean Average Precision (mAP) of 66%. Meanwhile RCNN, SPP-Net (Spatial Pyramid Pooling in Deep Convolutional Networks for Visual Recognition) has been introduced by (He et al., 2015) to refine recognition productivity. In the succession RESNET arrived to alleviate the problem of network migration with the incorporating residual module which also improves the depth of the network. Moreover it can obtain the features with stronger expression ability and higher accuracy (He et al., 2016). Multilayer Perceptron (MLP) is implemented to replace SVM are optimized significantly, which has been named as Fast RCNN (Girshick et al., 2014). In Fast RCNN, Ren S, He K, and Girshick upgraded RPN to select and modify the region proposals instead of selective search, which is aimed at solving the end-to-end detection problem; this is the Faster RCNN method. Liu Wei proposed a SSD (Single Shot MultiBox) method in ECCV2016 (EuropeanConference on Computer Vision; Ren et al., 2015). Compared with Faster RCNN, it hasa distinct speed advantage, which is able to directly predict the coordinates and categories of bounding box without processing of generating a proposal (Support Vector Machine); the training and classification.

The preceding section deals with the introduction to deep learning and fundamental architecture of CNN. The Faster RCNN-based object detection will be discussed in Section Three. Result analysis and future implementations are exhibited in Section Four.

5.2 CONVOLUTIONAL NEURAL NETWORK

The input layer is a collection of pixel intensities of RGB color channels in the form of three-dimensional matrixes. The specific feature of each pixel in the multichannel image is viewed in the feature map (Krizhevsky et al., 2017). Convolution and pooling operations are performed on the neurons with the activation function to deduce conclusive retaliation, as shown in Figure 5.2 (Oquab et al., 2014).

Visual perception assignment performed by an initial feature hierarchy constructed with the computations of convolution and pooling which can be further refined in a regulated in a smoother fashion by accumulating multiple Fully Connected (FC) layers. To obtain a conditional probability for every neuron, the last stage of the network is supplied with an activation function (Krizhevsky et al., 2017). It can be changed depending upon variations in the task. The entire network can be optimised through the Stochastic Gradient Descent (SGD) method using an objective function like MSE or cross-entropy loss (Oquab et al., 2014).

The standard VGG16 has a total of 13 convolution (conv) layers, three fully linked layers, three max pooling layers, and a classification layer of softmax. By convoluting 3*3 windows, convolution feature maps are created, and feature map resolutions are reduced with two-stride max pooling layers (Lecun et al., 2015). With a qualified network, arbitrary test pictures of the same size can be processed as training samples. If different sizes are given, rescaling or cropping may be necessary. CNN has several advantages over other methods, pointed out as follows. Striking capability is enhanced via the profound architecture of CNN.

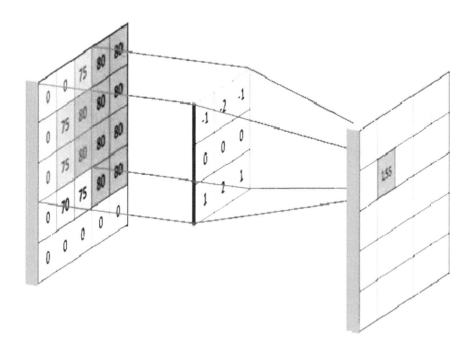

FIGURE 5.2   Convolution operation of CNN.

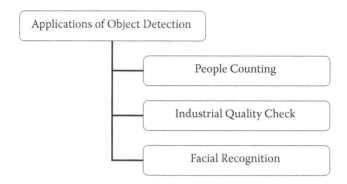

FIGURE 5.3 Few applications of object detection.

The architecture of CNN offers a way to combine and optimize many coherence jobs (e.g., Faster RCNN joins classification and regression together, which are incorporated in multi-task handling). Due to its advantages, CNN is widely used in a variety of research areas, such as image classification (Zeiler et al., 2010, Noh et al., 2015), image reconstruction (Zhao et al., 2014), video analytics (Babenko et al., 2014, Ngiam et al., 2011), image retrieval (Wan et al., 2014), pedestrian detection (Tomè et al., 2016) and face detection (Ngiam et al., 2011), as shown in Figure 5.3.

5.3 REGION PROPOSAL-BASED FRAMEWORK

RPN is a two-stage process. First RPN scans the object similar to the human attention to object and secondly drives its vision to the ROI (Zhao et al., 2019). RPN groups images as input and output in rectangular bounding boxes, each having an objectness score is defined to measure how well the detector identifies the locations and classes of objects during navigation (Szegedy et al., 2014), as shown in Figure 5.4. RPN initially produces a set of anchor boxes from the convolution feature map generated from the fundamental network. This links CNN to the sliding window method and identifies bounding boxes from locations of the pre-eminent feature map, once having acquired the confidence measure of objects to be detected (Long et al., 2015). Faster RCNN inherits a selective search algorithm to produce about 2,000 RPN per image (Nair, Hinton, 2010). The selective search method depends on reverse grouping and significant cues to instill more accurate candidate boxes of random sizes instantly and reduce search space in object detection (Ren et al., 2016).

After the creation of RPN, extensive features are extracted by wrapping or cropping with fixed resolution. CNN modules are incorporated to extract features with dimension of 4,096 as the conclusive representation. RCNN has vast learning capabilities; enormous power and defined structural representation aids in achieving robust feature representation for individual RPN. With the support of transfer learning (pre-trained category of weights), linear SVM's are utilized for multiple classification based on different RPN scores, which depict the positive

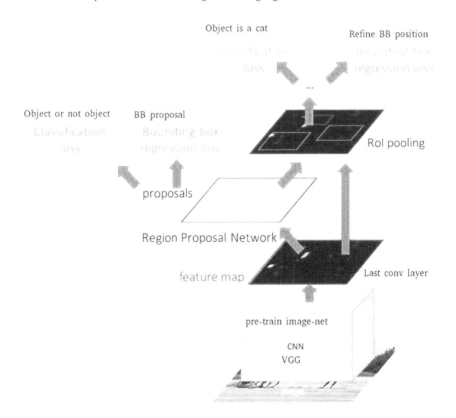

FIGURE 5.4   RPN module serves as the 'attention' of this unified network.

and background regions. The scores are refined with bounding boxes and suppressed by a greedy Non Maximum Suppression (NMS) to construct a precise bounding box to extract ROI and remove duplicates.

A sliding window is moved over the RPN's, where the quantity of proposals per location is k. The regression layers, having 4,000 outputs, represent the coordinates of k boxes. The classification layer outputs 2,000 scores, which estimates the probability of the object belonging to the proposal. The reference boxes (k numbers) are called anchors, and parameterize k proposals related to scale and aspect ratio, depicted in Figure 5.5.

Generally three aspect ratios and three scales are utilized for generating nine anchors for sliding, as shown in Figure 5.6. For a convolution feature map of a size W × H (say typically ~2,400), W Hk anchors would be generated (Szegedy et al., 2014).

The vital attribute of this approach is that it is translation invariant, both with respect to anchors and functions which claculate proposals relative to the anchors. If we consider the size of the original image as 800 × 600, VGG is downsampled 16 times and nine anchors are set for each point of the feature map, so: (800/16) × (600/16) × 9 = 50 × 38 × 9 results in 17,100 number of anchors, shown in Figure 5.7.

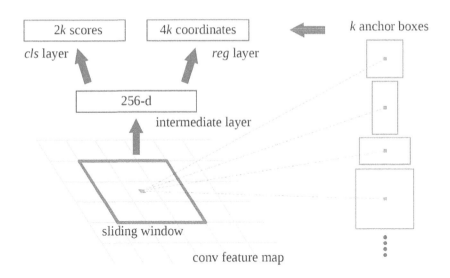

FIGURE 5.5   Regional proposal network.

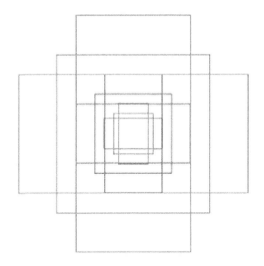

FIGURE 5.6   Anchors for sliding.

Softmax classifies the candidate box background image is positive or negative anchors, after the M × N-sized image is sent to the Faster RCNN network, the RPN network becomes (M/16) × (N/16) after convolution is W × H × 18. There are exactly 9 anchors for each point in the feature maps. At the same time, each anchor may be positive or negative. All this information is stored in a W × H × (9 × 2) size matrix. Later, the softmax classifies the positive anchors, that is, the box (in the positive anchors) of the preliminary detection target area is initially extracted. The matrix contains positive/negative anchors, are stored in the form of

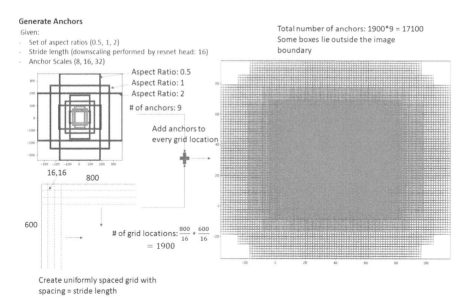

FIGURE 5.7   Total number of anchors generated.

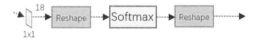

FIGURE 5.8   Softmax classification.

caffe blob with a size of [1, 2 × 9, H, W]. In the softmax classification as shown in Figure 5.8, a positive/negative binary classification is required, so the reshape layer will change it to a size of [1, 2, 9 × H, W]. That is, a dimension is vacated separately for softmax classification, and then reshape returns to its original state. In a nutshell, the RPN network uses anchors and softmax to initially extract positive anchors as candidate frames.

5.4   BOUNDING BOX REGRESSION PRINCIPLE

As shown in Figure 5.8, the green frame is the Ground Truth (GT) of mask detection and the red is the extracted positive anchors. If the red frame is recognized by the classifier as mask detection, but is not positioned correctly, the picture is equivalent to no mask. The mask was correctly detected. So it's vital to fine tune the red box to make positive anchors and the GT closer.

5.5   PROPOSAL LAYER

This layer is responsible for synthesizing all the transform amounts and positive anchors, calculating accurate proposals, and inputting them to the subsequent ROI Pooling Layer. Layers have three inputs: the classification results of positive

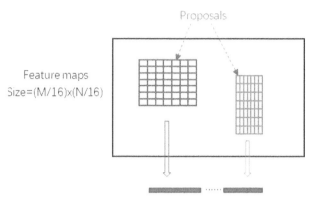

FIGURE 5.9   Calculating accurate proposals.

negative anchors; the corresponding box regression transformation amounts; and rpn_bbox_pred and im_info, and feat_stride = 16. As shown in Figure 5.9, im_info = [M, N, scale_factor = 1/16] holds all the scaling information for calculating offset of the anchor.

The steps behind proposal layer formation has given below:

1. Generate anchors, and use bbox regression for all anchors. (Generating anchors is exactly the same as training).
2. Sort the anchors in descending order according to the input positive scores, and extract the top N anchors; that is, extract the positive anchors after position correction.
3. Limit the image positive to the boundary of the image.
4. Remove very small (definite length and width) positive anchors.
5. Do NMS for the remaining positives.
6. The proposals layer has three inputs: the classification results of positive and negative anchors, and the corresponding bounding box regression results as the proper input.

The prime job of RoI pooling is to produce and aggregate the proposal, compute the proposal feature maps, and pass them to the predecessor network. From Figure 5.2 we can see that RoI pooling has two inputs:

1. Original feature maps.
2. Proposal boxes output by RPN.

For traditional CNN (VGG, ResNet), during training of network, the input image dimension must be a firm value and the network output must be a firm-size vector. If the input dimensions of the images are not the same, it becomes very troublesome. There are two methods to solve this:

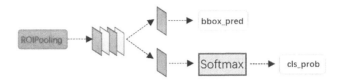

FIGURE 5.10   The classification network diagram.

1. Crop part from the image and transfer it to the network.
2. Warp the image to the required size.

It can be seen that no matter which method is adopted, either the complete structure of the image is destroyed after crop, or the original shape information of the image is destroyed by warp. RoI pooling alleviates the issue of how to deal with different sizes.

RoI Pooling works as follows:

The proposal corresponds to the M * N size; it is first mapped back to the size of the feature map (1/16) using the spatial_scale parameter. The feature map area corresponding to each proposal is divided into a grid; max_pooling is performed on each part of the grid.

After this processing, the output results of the proposals produce a fixed-length output as shown in Figure 5.10. The input of the classification part are the proposal feature maps, passed through the full connect layer. This then attains softmax to calculate which category each proposal belongs to and output of the cls_prob probability vector. Simultaneously, bbox regression obtains the position offset bbox_pred of each proposal, which returns accurate detection frame. The classification network diagram is shown below in Figure 5.10.

5.6   FASTER RCNN TRAINING

Faster RCNN continues to train from previously-trained models (VGG, resnet). In fact, the training process has the following six steps:

1. On the trained model, train the RPN network, corresponding to stage1_rpn_train.pt
2. Use the RPN network trained in step 1, collect proposals, corresponding to rpn_test.pt
3. First, train the Faster RCNN network twice, corresponding to stage1_fast_rcnn_train.pt
4. Train the RPN network twice, corresponding to stage2_rpn_train.pt
5. Use the RPN network trained in step four to collect the proposals, corresponding to rpn_test.pt
6. Train the Fast RCNN for once again corresponding to stage2_fast_rcnn_train.pt. The training process is similar to "iteration", and it is looped twice. A similar alternating training can be run for more iterations, but we have observed negligible improvements are shown in Figure 5.11.

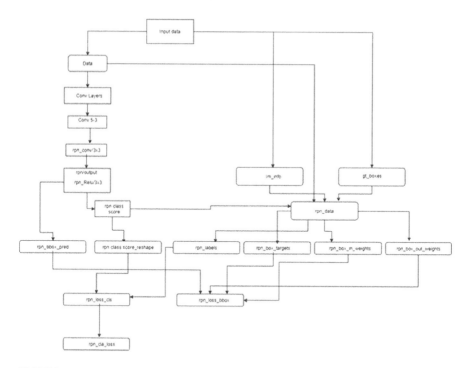

FIGURE 5.11 Overall working of faster RCNN.

The first step in finding the loss function in learning region proposals for RPNs is to designate every anchor as binary class (Szegedy et al., 2014). Next, a positive label is allocated to two types of anchors: (i) the anchor/anchors with the peak Intersection over-Union (IoU) which gets overlaid with a ground-truth box; or (ii) an anchor that has an IoU overlap greater than 0.7 with any ground-truth box (Girshick, 2015). A negative label is fixed to a negative anchor if its IoU ratio is less than 0.3 for all ground-truth boxes (He et al., 2015). Anchors which don't possess positive nor negative labels are ruled out for training. The loss function to minimize an objective function is given by

$$L(\{p_i\}, \{t_i\}) = \frac{1}{N_{cls}} \sum_i L_{cls}(p_i, p_i^*) + \frac{1}{N_{reg}} \sum_i p_i^* L_{reg}(t_i, t_i^*) \qquad (5.1)$$

"where i is the index representing an anchor in a mini batch and pi represents the predicted probability of an anchor. The ground-truth label, which p * i, has a value of one for a positive and zero for a negative. The ti vector signifies the four parameterized coordinates of the predicted bounding box, and t * i represents that the ground-truth box is associated with a positive anchor. The classification loss Lcls signifies the log loss over two classes (object vs. not object). Regression loss is represented by Lreg (ti, t* i) = R(ti − t * i), where R is the robust loss function (smooth L1) (Girshick, 2015). The term p * i Lreg represents the regression loss which will be activated only for positive anchors (p * i = 1). The output of the classification layer is comprised of {pi}, whereas the output of the regression layers is comprised of {ti}. Ncls and Nregs were the terminologies utilized for normalizing which has been weighted by a balancing parameter λ. In our present incorporation the classification term in equation (5.1) has been normalized by the mini-batch size (i.e., Ncls = 256) and the regression term is normalized by the number of anchor locations (i.e., Nreg ~ 2, 400). We have chosen default λ = 10 as balancing para-meter so that both classification and regression terms were equally weighted. For bounding box regression, we adopt the parameterizations of the four coordinates as shown in equation (5.2) (Girshick et al., 2014):

$$t_x = \frac{x - x_a}{w_a}, \qquad t_y = \frac{y - y_a}{h_a}$$
$$t_w = \log\left(\frac{w}{w_a}\right), \quad t_h = \log\left(\frac{h}{h_a}\right)$$
$$t_x^* = \frac{x - x_a}{w_a}, \qquad t_y^* = \frac{y - y_a}{h_a} \qquad (5.2)$$
$$t_w^* = \log\left(\frac{w^*}{w_a}\right), \quad t_h^* = \log\left(\frac{h^*}{h_a}\right)$$

X, y, w, and h represent the box's mid-coordinates, width and height. Variables x, xa, and x * signify the predicted box, anchor box, and ground truth box respectively. This method accomplishes bounding-box regression by a contrasting manner from previous RoI-based (Region of Interest) methods (He et al., 2015, Girshick, 2015). In (Szegedy et al., 2014, Girshick, 2015), bounding-box regression was conducted on features which were pooled from arbitrarily-sized RoIs and the regression weights were staked by all region sizes. In order to tackle the dynamic sizes, a set of k bounding-box regressors was learned. All the regressors contribute one scale and one aspect ratio. During this contribution the regressors do not share their weights (Du et al., 2017). Due to this feature it has the ability to predict boxes of various sizes though the features are of a fixed size/scale.

The closs softmax network, used to classify anchors as positive and negative networks and Reg loss (L1 loss), is calculated by the rpnlossbbox layer which has been used for bbox regression network training. In synopsis, the extracted proposals are transferred to the network as ROI and bbox_inside_weights + bbox_outside_-weights are calculated then passed into the soomth_L1_loss layer. As shown in the green box in Figure 5.12, it trains the final softmax and the final bbox regression.

5.7   NEED OF GPU CLOUD

Computer vision-based tasks are computationally exhaustive and monotonous, which overwhelms the capabilities of a CPU. In replacement, there was a technological transformation to Graphical Processing Unit (GPU) which envisioned the task of computer vision algorithms (Nguyen, 2019). Its data streaming and aggressive parallel processing architecture makes GPU suitable for computer vision processing. GPU accelerates computer vision tasks and the CPU can be used for other operations. Multiple GPU's can be used in a single machine to enhance the capability of multiple

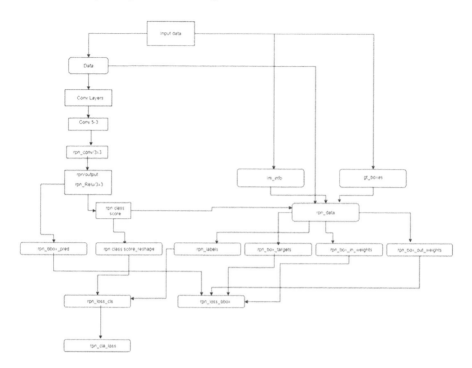

FIGURE 5.12 Flowchart of faster RCNN.

vision algorithms in parallel. Many GPU's are available in the market; popular ones are OpenGL and Nvidia (Sunnyvale,CA,USA; www.sgi.com). The Nvidia Compute Unified Device Architecture (CUDA) imparts a number of extensions to the C language, which allows programmers to send portions of their source code for execution on the device (https://www.cdac.in/index.aspx?id=ev_hpc_gpu-comp-nvidia-cudaprog-overview). Nvidia delivers a host, device and common component runtime along CUDA to incubate and supervise the computations on the GPU, eliminating the requirement to map them to a graphics API. While programming via CUDA, the GPU is regarded as a computation device able to execute a number of threads in parallel, and allows compute-intensive sections of applications executing on the host to be offloaded onto the GPU. Obviously GPUs are famously expensive – high-end Nvidia Teslas can be priced well above $10,000. To overcome this bottleneck, cloud services are provided by AWS, Paperspace, GCP, and cloud. Among them Paperspace provides comparatively economical, high-processing and thunderstorm GPU cloud sevices. Paperspace holds a free cloud GPU service for machine/deep learning development on the company's cloud computing and deep-learning platform. Designed for students and professionals learning how to build, train and deploy machine-learning models, the service can be thought of as an ML/DL starter kit that helps developers expand their skills and try out new ideas without financial risk (https://tensorflow.rstudio.com/installation/gpu/cloud_desktop_gpu/)

Besides access to free GPUs and CPUs, Paperspace and Gradient Community Notebooks offer a Jupyter-based collaborative environment, access to popular libraries, prebuilt models, and a project showcase, and allow users to create a public profile page to share their bio and the work they're interested in. Users can start from scratch with a new notebook or leverage pre-configured projects from the Gradient ML-Showcase, a curated list of machine-learning examples. One of the products of Paperspace is Gradient which, disentangles developing, training, and deploying deep- learning models. The platform provides infrastructure automation and a software development kit for machine-learning developers. In this work, we deployed our computer vision algorithm for mask detection using Paperspace cloud services. Though Paperspace provides free services with limited editions, we didn't meet the requirements. We rented a machine Ubuntu 18.04 Desktop MLiab, with P4000 hourly at a cost of $7/month+/ hour of usage per month for months.

5.8   TENSORFLOW OBJECT DETECTION (TFOD)

The object detection model can distinguish known sets of objects present in an image or video; it also provides information about positions. This model detects the existence of numerous classes of objects. Confidence of detection is scored from 0 to 1. This score reveals the confidence of detection gathered from the location of the bounding box which contains each object. TFOD API is a framework for constructing a deep-learning network that decodes object detection, utilizing the pre-trained models available in the model zoo. It can be used for training a naïve dataset; various architectures available in the model zoo are tabulated in Table 5.1.

TABLE 5.1
COCO pre-trained models in model zoo

Model name	Speed (ms)	COCO mAP	Outputs
CenterNet HourGlass104 512x512	70	41.9	Boxes
CenterNet HourGlass104 Keypoints 512x512	76	40.0/61.4	Boxes/Keypoints
CenterNet HourGlass104 1024x1024	197	44.5	Boxes
CenterNet HourGlass104 Keypoints 1024x1024	211	42.8/64.5	Boxes/Keypoints
CenterNet Resnet50 V1 FPN 512x512	27	31.2	Boxes
CenterNet Resnet50 V1 FPN Keypoints 512x512	30	29.3/50.7	Boxes/Keypoints
CenterNet Resnet101 V1 FPN 512x512	34	34.2	Boxes
CenterNet Resnet50 V2 512x512	27	29.5	Boxes
CenterNet Resnet50 V2 Keypoints 512x512	30	27.6/48.2	Boxes/Keypoints
EfficientDet D0 512x512	39	33.6	Boxes
EfficientDet D1 640x640	54	38.4	Boxes
EfficientDet D2 768x768	67	41.8	Boxes
EfficientDet D3 896x896	95	45.4	Boxes
EfficientDet D4 1024x1024	133	48.5	Boxes
EfficientDet D5 1280x1280	222	49.7	Boxes
EfficientDet D6 1280x1280	268	50.5	Boxes

(Continued)

TABLE 5.1 (Continued)

Model name	Speed (ms)	COCO mAP	Outputs
EfficientDet D7 1536x1536	325	51.2	Boxes
SSD MobileNet v2 320x320	19	20.2	Boxes
SSD MobileNet V1 FPN 640x640	48	29.1	Boxes
SSD MobileNet V2 FPNLite 320x320	22	22.2	Boxes
SSD MobileNet V2 FPNLite 640x640	39	28.2	Boxes
SSD ResNet50 V1 FPN 640x640 (RetinaNet50)	46	34.3	Boxes
SSD ResNet50 V1 FPN 1024x1024 (RetinaNet50)	87	38.3	Boxes
SSD ResNet101 V1 FPN 640x640 (RetinaNet101)	57	35.6	Boxes
SSD ResNet101 V1 FPN 1024x1024 (RetinaNet101)	104	39.5	Boxes
SSD ResNet152 V1 FPN 640x640 (RetinaNet152)	80	35.4	Boxes
SSD ResNet152 V1 FPN 1024x1024 (RetinaNet152)	111	39.6	Boxes
Faster R-CNN ResNet50 V1 640x640	53	29.3	Boxes
Faster R-CNN ResNet50 V1 1024x1024	65	31.0	Boxes
Faster R-CNN ResNet50 V1 800x1333	65	31.6	Boxes
Faster R-CNN ResNet101 V1 640x640	55	31.8	Boxes
Faster R-CNN ResNet101 V1 1024x1024	72	37.1	Boxes
Faster R-CNN ResNet101 V1 800x1333	77	36.6	Boxes
Faster R-CNN ResNet152 V1 640x640	64	32.4	Boxes
Faster R-CNN ResNet152 V1 1024x1024	85	37.6	Boxes
Faster R-CNN ResNet152 V1 800x1333	101	37.4	Boxes
Faster R-CNN Inception ResNet V2 640x640	206	37.7	Boxes
Faster R-CNN Inception ResNet V2 1024x1024	236	38.7	Boxes
Mask R-CNN Inception ResNet V2 1024x1024	301	39.0/34.6	Boxes/Masks
ExtremeNet	–	–	Boxes

5.9 CONFIGURATION STEPS FOR TENSOR FLOW OBJECT DETECTION

Configuration steps for tensor flow object detection is given below as shown in https://c17hawke.github.io/tfod-setup/

5.10 RESULTS AND ANALYSIS

The frozen model generates a unique file holding all details regarding graph and checkpoint variables; it also holds the information of hyper- parameters as constants inside the graph structure. This eliminates additional information saved in check-point files, such as the gradients of each point, which are included so that the model can be reloaded and training continued from where you left off. The above procedure was repeated twice; to obtain the person-detection frozen graph. we used

Single Shot Detection Lite. The second frozen graph was obtained for mask detection, which utilized Faster RCNN algorithm.

The frozen graphs were transferred from GPU to a local system, to detect masks and social distance. We used pycharm 2020 community edition as the platform, with python version 3.6.9. Initially we created a conda environment named mask_detect and activated it. To execute this program, many library files need to be installed; hence, all required packages were packed in a single file as requirements.txt, which was installed by executing the command conda install –r requirements.txt.

A tensorflow session was created and the frozen graph, which was transferred from GPU to CPU, was loaded. In the program Opencv, the package was used to activate the camera to receive video input. Bounding boxes were drawn for detecting people. If people were detected, bounding boxes were drawn to detect if the person was wearing a mask. After successful detection of a person wearing a mask, the distance between two people was computed by the bounding boxes by drawing a virtual line. If social distance was not maintained, an alert would sound. The following figures depict the results of the study. Figure 5.13 shows a person with a mask. SSD mobilenet detects the person whereas Faster RCNN detects the person without a mask and produces a beep signal along with an alert image. Figure 5.14 detects the person wearing a mask. Figure 5.15 shows multiple persons with masks; an alert signal is produced since they haven't maintained social distance (distance is calculated between two bounding boxes; accordingly, the distance has been changed from 2.5 m to 2.0 m in order to extract the exact distance between persons). An alert signal is produced in Figure 5.15, even though the persons are wearing masks, since they aren't maintaining social distance. In Figure 5.16, two people are not wearing masks, nor is social distance maintained, so an alert signal is produced. In Figure 5.17, an alert signal is not produced since the people are wearing masks and maintaining social distance.

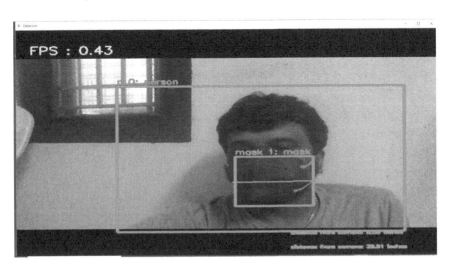

FIGURE 5.13 Person with mask.

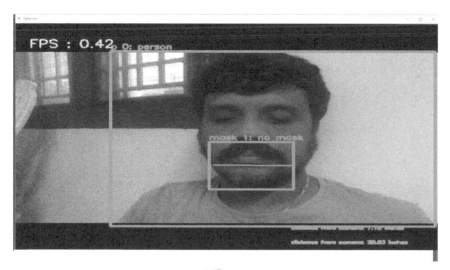

FIGURE 5.14 Person without mask.

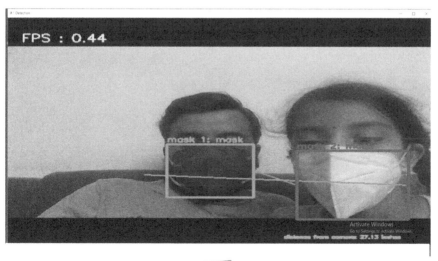

FIGURE 5.15 Persons wearing masks and neglecting social distance.

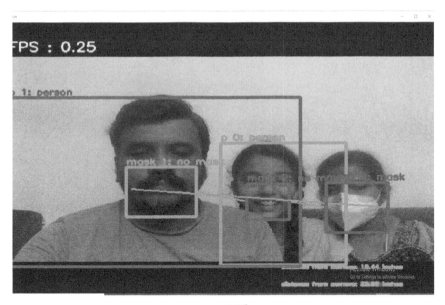

FIGURE 5.16   Mixed people neglecting social distance.

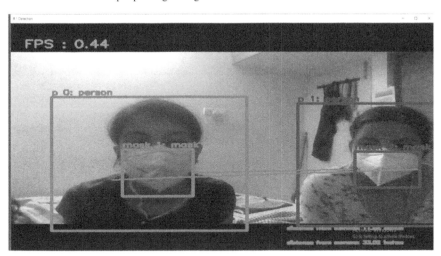

FIGURE 5.17   People wearing masks and maintaining social distance.

5.11   CONCLUSION AND FUTURE SCOPE

The major focus of this study is face mask and social distancing detection, and methods to give warning if they are not followed. To meet real-time requirements for person detection, we designed SSD Mobilenet lite, and for mask detection, the Faster RCNN algorithm. Based on these algorithms, image recognition, detection and segmentation were improved, which we can conclude from the figures. The network formed by Faster RCNN and Mobile SSD lite, accurately detects a distance of about 30m in different light conditions. This network can be applied for mask detection and warning if a person is not wearing a mask or maintaining social distance.

In future work, we aim to include thermal cameras, which can detect body temperature efficiently (as compared with infrared thermometers) and reduce the work and improve the safety of security personnel. To make it viable, we are planning to use Fluke Connect thermal cameras to measure body temperature. We are in the process of automating thermals camera by incorporating computer vision methods, so that 100% automatic detection will result. This will be a beneficial tool for accessing and monitoring students after the lifting of lockdown.

REFERENCES

Babenko, A., Slesarev, A., Chigorin, A., & Lempitsky, V. (2014, September). Neural codes for image retrieval. In *European Conference on Computer Vision* (pp. 584–599). Springer, Cham.

Dai, J., Li, Y., He, K., & Sun, J. (2016). R-fcn: Object detection via region-based fully convolutional networks. *Advances in Neural Information Processing Systems*, *29*, 379–387.

Deng, J., Dong, W., Socher, R., Li, L. J., Li, K., & Fei-Fei, L. (2009, June). Imagenet: A large-scale hierarchical image database. In *2009 IEEE Conference on Computer Vision and Pattern Recognition* (pp. 248–255). IEEE.

Du, X., El-Khamy, M., Lee, J., & Davis, L. (2017, March). Fused DNN: A deep neural network fusion approach to fast and robust pedestrian detection. In *2017 IEEE Winter Conference on Applications of Computer Vision (WACV)* (pp. 953–961). IEEE.

Erhan, D., Szegedy, C., Toshev, A., & Anguelov, D. (2014). Scalable object detection using deep neural networks. In Proceedings of the *IEEE Conference on Computer Vision and Pattern Recognition* (pp. 2147–2154).

Ghosh, A., Nundy, S., & Mallick, T. K. (2020). How India is dealing with COVID-19 pandemic. *Sensors International*, *1*, 100021.

Girshick, R. (2015). Fast r-cnn. In *Proceedings of the IEEE International Conference on Computer Vision* (pp. 1440–1448).

Girshick, R., Donahue, J., Darrell, T., & Malik, J. (2014). Rich feature hierarchies for accurate object detection and semantic segmentation. In Proceedings of the *IEEE Conference on Computer Vision and Pattern Recognition* (pp. 580–587).

Gopalan, H. S., Misra, A. (2020). COVID-19 pandemic and challenges for socio-economic issues, healthcare and National Health Programs in India. *Diabetes & Metabolic Syndrome: Clinical Research & Reviews*, *14*, 757–759, https://doi.org/10.1016/j.dsx.2 020.05.041.

He, K., Zhang, X., Ren, S., & Sun, J. (2015). Spatial pyramid pooling in deep convolutional networks for visual recognition. *IEEE Transactions on Pattern Analysis and Machine Intelligence*, *37*(9), 1904–1916.

He, K., Zhang, X., Ren, S., & Sun, J. (2016). Deep residual learning for image recognition. In *Proceedings of the IEEE Conference on Computer Vision and Pattern Recognition* (pp. 770–778).

He, K., Gkioxari, G., Doll´ar, P., & Girshick, R. B. (2017) Mask r-cnn, In Proceedings of the IEEE International Conference on Computer Vision, *1*(6), 2961–2969.

https://www.hindustantimes.com/education/unlock-4-schools-across-india-reopen-partially-from-today/story-PitHi6Wwvy7eknOfMpCKJK.html.

Huang, R., Pedoeem, J., & Chen, C. (2018, December). YOLO-LITE: a real-time object detection algorithm optimized for non-GPU computers. In *2018 IEEE International Conference on Big Data (Big Data)* (pp. 2503–2510). IEEE.

Indian Council of Medical Research (2020). Press Release ICMR Process to Develop Vaccine to Fight Covid 19 Pandemic as Per Globally Accepted Norms of Fast Tracking Safety and Interest of People of India the Topmost Priority.

Krizhevsky A., Sutskever I., Hinton G. E. (2012) Imagenet classification with deep convolutional neural networks. In *Proceedings of the 25th international conference on neural information processing systems - volume 1, NIPS'12*, (pp. 1097–1105). Curran Associates Inc., Red Hook, NY, USA.

Krizhevsky, A., Sutskever, I., & Hinton, G. E. (2017). Imagenet classification with deep convolutional neural networks. *Communications of the ACM, 60*(6), 84–90.

Lecun Y., Bengio Y., Hinton G. (2015a) Deep learning. *Nature Cell Biology, 521*(7553), 436–444.

LeCun, Y., Bengio, Y., & Hinton, G. (2015b). Deep learning. *Nature, 521*(7553), 436–444.

Lin, T. Y., Dollár, P., Girshick, R., He, K., Hariharan, B., & Belongie, S. (2017). Feature pyramid networks for object detection. In *Proceedings of the IEEE Conference on Computer Vision and Pattern Recognition* (pp. 2117–2125).

Liu, W., Anguelov, D., Erhan, D., Szegedy, C., Reed, S., Fu, C. Y., & Berg, A. C. (2016, October). Ssd: Single shot multibox detector. In *European conference on computer vision* (pp. 21–37). Springer, Cham.

Long, J., Shelhamer, E., & Darrell, T. (2015). Fully convolutional networks for semantic segmentation. In Proceedings of the *IEEE Conference on Computer Vision and Pattern Recognition* (pp. 3431–3440).

Mahato, S., Pal, S., & Ghosh, K. G. (2020). Effect of lockdown amid COVID-19 pandemic on air quality of the megacity Delhi, India. *Science of the Total Environment, 730*, 139086.

Mehta K., & Jha, S. S. (2020). COVID-19: A nightmare for the Indian economy. *UGC Care Journal, 31*(20), 333–347. https://doi.org/10.2139/ssrn.3612676

Nair, V., & Hinton, G. E. (2010, January). Rectified linear units improve restricted boltzmann machines, In International Conference on Machine Learning, 807–814.

Najibi, M., Rastegari, M., & Davis, L. S. (2016). G-cnn: an iterative grid based object detector. In Proceedings of the *IEEE Conference on Computer Vision and Pattern Recognition* (pp. 2369–2377).

Ngiam, J., Khosla, A., Kim, M., Nam, J., Lee, H., & Ng, A. Y. (2011, January). Multimodal deep learning, In International Conference on Machine Learning, 689–696.

Nguyen, H. (2019). Improving faster R-CNN framework for fast vehicle detection. *Mathematical Problems in Engineering, 2019*, 1–11.

Nieto-Rodríguez, A., Mucientes, M., & Brea, V. M. (2015, September). Mask and maskless face classification system to detect breach protocols in the operating room. In Proceedings of the *9th International Conference on Distributed Smart Cameras* (pp. 207–208).

Noh, H., Hong, S., & Han, B. (2015). Learning deconvolution network for semantic segmentation. In Proceedings of the *IEEE International Conference on Computer Vision* (pp. 1520–1528).

Oquab, M., Bottou, L., Laptev, I., & Sivic, J. (2014). Learning and transferring mid-level image representations using convolutional neural networks. In Proceedings of the *IEEE conference on computer vision and pattern recognition* (pp. 1717–1724).

Redmon, J., & Farhadi, A. (2017). YOLO9000: better, faster, stronger. In Proceedings of the *IEEE Conference on Computer Vision and Pattern Recognition* (pp. 7263–7271).

Redmon, J., & Farhadi, A. (2018). Yolov3: An incremental improvement. *arXiv preprint arXiv:1804.02767.*

Ren, S., He, K., Girshick, R., & Sun, J. (2016). Faster R-CNN: Towards real-time object detection with region proposal networks. *IEEE Transactions on Pattern Analysis and Machine Intelligence*, *39*(6), 1137–1149.

Roy, B., Nandy, S., Ghosh, D., Dutta, D., Biswas, P., & Das, T. (2020). MOXA: A deep learning based unmanned approach for real-time monitoring of people wearing medical masks. *Transactions of the Indian National Academy of Engineering*, *5*(3), 509–518.

Szegedy, C., Reed, S., Erhan, D., Anguelov, D., & Ioffe, S. (2014). Scalable, high-quality object detection. *arXiv preprint arXiv:1412.1441.*

Szegedy, C., Vanhoucke, V., Ioffe, S., Shlens, J., & Wojna, Z. (2016) Rethinking the inception architecture for computer vision. In *2016 IEEE Conference on Computer Vision and Pattern Recognition (CVPR).*

Tomè, D., Monti, F., Baroffio, L., Bondi, L., Tagliasacchi, M., & Tubaro, S. (2016). Deep convolutional neural networks for pedestrian detection. *Signal Processing: Image Communication*, *47*, 482–489.

Uijlings, J., van de Sande, K.E.A., Gevers, T., & Smeulders, A. W. M. (2013). Selective search for object recognition, *International Journal of Computer Vision*, *104*(2), 154–171.

Viola, Paul, Michael J., J. (2004). Robust real-time face detection, *International Journal of Computer Vision*, *57*(2), 137–154.

Wan, J., Wang, D., Hoi, S. C. H., Wu, P., Zhu, J., Zhang, Y., & Li, J. (2014, November). Deep learning for content-based image retrieval: A comprehensive study. In Proceedings of the *22nd ACM International Conference on Multimedia* (pp. 157–166).

Wu, Z., Wang, X., Jiang, Y. G., Ye, H., & Xue, X. (2015, October). Modeling spatial-temporal clues in a hybrid deep learning framework for video classification. In Proceedings of the *23rd ACM international conference on Multimedia* (pp. 461–470).

Yoo, D., Park, S., Lee, J. Y., Paek, A. S., & So Kweon, I. (2015). Attentionnet: Aggregating weak directions for accurate object detection. In Proceedings of the *IEEE International Conference on Computer Vision* (pp. 2659–2667).

Zeiler, M. D., Krishnan, D., Taylor, G. W., & Fergus, R. (2010, June). Deconvolutional networks. In *2010 IEEE Computer Society Conference on Computer Vision and Pattern Recognition* (pp. 2528–2535). IEEE.

Zhao, Z. Q., Xie, B. J., Cheung, Y. M., & Wu, X. (2014, November). Plant leaf identification via a growing convolution neural network with progressive sample learning. In *Asian Conference on Computer Vision* (pp. 348–361). Springer, Cham.

Zhao, Z. Q., Zheng, P., Xu, S. T., & Wu, X. (2019). Object detection with deep learning: A review. *IEEE Transactions on Neural Networks and Learning Systems*, *30*(11), 3212–3232.

6 Review of Effective Mathematical Modelling of Coronavirus Epidemic and Effect of drone Disinfection

Agnishwar Jayaprakash[1], R. Nithya[2], and M. Kayalvizhi[2]
[1]Agni Foundation, Chennai, India
[2]Department of Biomedical Engineering, Agni College of Technology, Chennai, India

6.1 INTRODUCTION

COVID-19 (coronavirus disease 2019) is a catastrophe which has taken numerous lives and is a worldwide concern. Coronavirus causes a serious intense respiratory instability, sometimes leading to death. It has affected over 41 lakhs of individuals and killed practically 28 lakhs individuals worldwide. Hence, the World Health Organization (WHO) has proclaimed it an international pandemic. Currently, it does not have a viable immunization or treatment method [Ayittey F. K; 2020, Yang Y; 2020a, Winter G; 2020, Zhu S; 2020]. It has dangerous impacts, particularly in people with less immunity. The onset of COVID-19 has hindered socioeconomic and commercial activity throughout the world [Luo, G; 2020, Foster K. A; 2020, Wang P; 2020]. With concerns existing around the pandemic, there is a need to restrict the spread of infection [Carinci F; 2020, Ji S; 2020, Lee Y; 2016, Li Y; 2017, Yang Y; 2020, Fiorillo L; 2020, Cavallo L; 2020, Colson P; 2016]. The epidemic spreads mainly through respiratory droplets, and direct contact with infected people or surfaces. The virus lives on public surfaces for various periods of time; it can be inactivated easily, by utilizing chemical disinfectants. Indian cities have taken substantial measures to decontaminate major urban communities, particularly high-risk public spaces. Urban communities are using various ways to deal with cleaning public spaces, including transport terminals, railroad stations, markets, and so on [Cohen J; 2020, Li X; 2020, Zhang S; 2011, Rodriguez-Morales A; 2020, Wood C; 2020, Azamfirei R; 2020, Watts C; 2020, Khan S; 2020, Murdoch D; 2020].

Urban communities are adopting creative strategies for decontaminating public spots using laborers. These procedures are difficult when used consistently, and tiring for the laborers. It is additionally found to cause dermatological and allergic reactions in the laborers. Urban communities are adopting new strategies for cleansing of public spots utilizing sodium hypochlorite. Disinfectant is sprayed in all parts of the city to protect it from any sort of contamination. Sanitation laborers spray the disinfectant. Sterilization of an entire city is done with fogging, anti-larval spraying and disinfectant spraying [Cheshmehzangi A; 2020, Hansen S; 2018, Thompson-Dyk K; 2016, Yang W; 2017, Romantsov M.G; 2010, Bloom G; 2015, Chen P; 2019, Schwerdtle P; 2017]. City administrations have guaranteed purification of all open spots in cities utilizing jetting machines. Vehicles and laborers can do only ground cleansing. Our cities have many apartments and high-rises with numerous floors; these are accessed using recent drone innovations. Recent innovations and independent machines are assuming a leading role in reacting to the COVID-19 pandemic. Be that as it may, in this battle against this imperceptible adversary, drones assume a vital part by helping specialists and individuals in various manners to forestall the spread of COVID-19. COVID-19 is a widespread health crisis of intercontinental concern. Currently there is no powerful drug treatment. This is an utmost requirement for treating those with the sickness.

The COVID-19 is profoundly contagious. The Centers for Disease Control and Prevention assessed that the infection's using a Reproduction number R0. It measures the number of secondary infected subjects that probably result from the existing virus infected cases and is in the range of 1.6 and 2.4. The corona virus is highly contagious disease and has a reproduction number between 1.2 and 1.4. The Mckinsey investigation shows casualties can be decreased by taking appropriate measures and giving legitimate treatment [Tahir R.F; 2020, Suroyo G; 2020]. Although R0 is basic for infectious prevention, It doesn't depict the level of reality of a sickness. The number of affected individuals who eventually die due to the ailment is called the casualty rate. Profoundly-communicable illnesses like measles, with a mean R0 of 15, have a relatively low case casualty rate. But for Ebola, 60% of patients die of the infection and Ro is low. Early evaluation rates demonstrate that the case casualty rate of COVID-19 is lower [Ji W; 2020, Benvenuto D; 2020, Liu Z; 2020, Lam T; 2020, Li X; 2020, Salata C; 2019, Malik; 2020]. It is found that case casualty rates are not constant; they rely heavily upon mitigation measures taken by the general public. The existing techniques that help to combat suffering due to serious intense respiratory symptoms of COVID-19 (SARS-CoV-2) are decreasing transmission of the virus by cleaning and social distancing. The Mckinsey report shows the essential mode of transmission of the infection is the presence of the virus in the air, which remains for around three hours. It also spreads in surfaces like cardboard, paper, glasses, metals, wood, plastics, ceramics and stone. It normally persists on these surfaces for four days. Hence, by disinfecting the surfaces and structures around us, we curb the current pandemic. However, the current disinfecting methods are tedious [GEN; 2020].

Drones can fly up to 150 meters and access buildings 400 feet high. During a pandemic, drones offer a helping hand to clean surfaces quickly. They help limit human intervention in curbing viral transmission [Kummitha R; 2020, Bannister F;

2020, Calvo R; 2020]. Drones can likewise be utilized to cover distant regions more effectively and rapidly than standard methods of disinfection [Li C; 2020, Huang J; 2020]. Tech pioneers and health care divisions are joining hands to use inventive approaches like drones to battle COVID-19 [Kharpal A; 2020, Power B; 2020].

Urban areas that took such mitigation steps had lower death and mortality rates. The current pandemic has made life miserable. There is a need for mathematical models to evaluate and study how an infection spreads. In India, where a large population has less immunity, nearly all affected individuals are contagious. The commonly-used model to represent this is the deterministic model [Li W; 2020]. Mathematical modelling has provided a reasonable means to perceive transmission progress of disease, as well as the proficiency to choose the most effective and economical interventions aimed at prevention and treatment.

6.2 METHODOLOGY

The worldwide spread of the pandemic, taking into account diverse people with dissimilar features, is modelled with limited significant features pertinent to the infection [Allen E; 2008, Raza A; 2019, Allen E; 2009, Arif M; 2019, Ekanayake; 2010, Bayram; 2018, Yuan Y; 2011]. The population is partitioned into compartments: communities susceptible to the disease; the disease-ridden; healed subjects; and immune subjects. The different subclasses of the population are termed compartments. In this model the individuals are categorized into compartments, depending on the ailment under study [Mollison D; 1995]. Further in this model, an individual in a population can be in one and only one compartment. It is possible for individuals to shift from one compartment to another depending on their status. In this chapter, we study SIR and SCIR compartment models. The simplest is the Susceptible-Infected-Recovered (SIR) model. In the SIR model, the whole population is sub-classed into susceptible(S), infected(I) and recovered(R) subjects. It helps foretell the contagious propagation of the pandemic. In this work, we offer a case study of disinfecting the city of Varanasi using drones. We also study the spread of disease using SIR mathematical model. In this deterministic model, contagious propagation of infection in the city is analysed using mathematical differential equations [McCluskey C; 2010]. In the population, the numbers of susceptible individuals $S(t)$ and infected individuals $I(t)$ in the given time t are considered. We assume that the rate of newly-infected individuals depends on both the count of infected and susceptible individuals. The equation is given by

$$I(t + \nabla t) = I(t) + \beta I(t)S(t)\nabla t \qquad (6.1)$$

Here β refers to the infection rate; it often also refers to the contact rate. Assumptions made in this mathematical model are that the removal parameter includes infected individuals with a chance of being quarantined, those who passed away or recovered, and those who were resistant with high immunity. The resistant or recovered individuals are eliminated and go to a new unsusceptible compartment.

The individuals who are removed a t time t from a compartment is given as $R(t)$ and γ is represented as removal rate. The equation is given as:

$$I(t) + S(t) + R(t) = n \qquad (6.2)$$

Here n represents the population size. The measures of the three quantities are given by the differential equations. Once the infected individuals are quarantined from the population, the susceptible individuals' chance of getting infected will be reduced. The count of individuals in the susceptible compartment at any time depends on exposure to infected individuals and the count of already existing susceptible individuals, as is represented in equation (6.3).

$$\frac{dS(t)}{dt} = -\beta S(t)I(t) \qquad (6.3)$$

In the case of infected individuals, the removal rate has to be considered in the formation of the differential equation. It can be obtained by modifying the equation (6.2).

$$\frac{dI}{dt} = \beta S(t)I(t) - \gamma I(t) \qquad (6.4)$$

Finally the differential equation governing the rate of removal depends on infected individuals from the population with removal rate γ; this is represented in equation (6.5).

$$\frac{dR(t)}{dt} = \gamma I(t) \qquad (6.5)$$

β in the equation is the transmission parameter. It signifies the mean of the subjects that one infected subject shall spread in the given time, with assumption that acquaintances was created by infected subject with susceptible subject. Higher β indicates that the disease is highly infectious. The parameter γ signifies the rate of recovery. The mean time a diseased subject remains affected is represented by $1/\gamma$. Further, the part of the community that will be infected per unitof time can be obtained using the product of $\beta S(t)$. The total infection rate is represented by I(t). In a city let us consider I(t) as the fraction of the community infected presently; they are in contact with all susceptible subjects of the community. There is a possibility of passing the infection to a proportion of $\beta I(t)$ community in the given time. In reality, only a proportion of S(t) of the community are in contact with infected people; they are susceptible presently and the possibility exists of infecting $\beta I(t)$ S(t) in the given time. The significant measure that quantifies the spread of pathogens is the basic reproductive number R0, given as the ratio β/γ [Zhou F; 2020]. Every pathogen that enters an individual has a infectivity period. The mean of people infected due to a diseased subject during the pathogenic period, in a completely susceptible community is given as R0. This simple SIR model helps provide some prominent predictions. The above differential equations are entered in Matlab, for the numerical solution of differential equations. β and γ collectively with S(0), I(0), and R(0) are initialised. Corresponding to this model, an epidemic curve of the considered city population is created. The curve estimates the proportion of the community that will be diseased in a particular period of pandemic study. The most important outcome of the model is the epidemic threshold Eth. It is the product of S(0) and R0. If Eth < 1, there will be no epidemic; the proportion of diseased subjects will promptly diminish. Further, if S(0) R0 > 1, there is a chance for the pandemic to spread and does not bother about the small initial proportion of the diseased individuals. The size of the pandemic tends to rely on the initial fraction of those susceptible, S(0), and on R0 when it occurs. It is not possible to rely on the initial count of infected. The proportion of the community infected, the size of the epidemic, has to be limited to the initial proportion of the community that was susceptible, S(0). Hence, the remaining a part of community of susceptible subjects is always not infected. The epidemic threshold also implies that, if measures are taken to keep the pathogen from spreading, it reduces the initial proportion of susceptible to S(0) < γ /β. Then we can avert the epidemic. In the proposed work we are trying to reduce the transmissibility parameter β by disinfecting public places with drones and studying the spread of the disease. Chlorine-based disinfectant spray is proved by WHO and other renowned virology institutes to kill 99% of bacteria and viruses.

A recent WHO news update shows that carriers without any symptoms are spreading the virus unknowingly. Asymptomatic diseased subjects were spotted, quarantined and kept under observation for the duration of the incubation period of 14 days. The Mckinsely report found that 20-50% are asymptomatic. Viral shedding of infected people lasts ten to 20 days. The case fatality ratio varies depending on measures taken by the government and people in different regions. Recently it was found the novel coronavirus undergoes an asymptomatic period at the beginning of the disease. During this time, these carriers can harbour the virus and spread the disease to their fellow beings without exhibiting symptoms. Hence, there is a requirement to include another compartment of subjects to the considered model. Such individuals, once afflicted, are proficient in transmitting the infection without exhibiting symptoms. They are the "carrier" compartment. Hence, S-I-R model is changed to S-C-I-R model [Sari E; 2019]. The carrier compartment is essential for the spread of the disease. Even the most accurate mathematical models need assumptions. Further, while considering small a community for study, the probability element has to be considered, and so stochastic models are selected. Recently it was found the novel coronavirus undergoes an asymptomatic period at the beginning of the disease. In the course of this time, these carrier can harbour the virus and spread the disease to their fellow being without exhibiting any symptoms. Hence there is a requirement to include another compartment to the model. The considered individuals, once afflicted, are contagious enough to spread the infection without any symptoms are the "carrier" class. Hence S-I-R model is changed to S-C-I-R model. The considered carrier compartment is essential to be considered because they spread the infection. Even the most accurate mathematical models are not Competent enough to predict the current pandemic. Mathematical modelling has

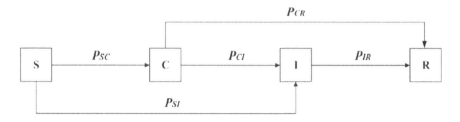

FIGURE 6.1 SCIR model of the disease.

played a great role in handling severe epidemics [Allen; 2008, Huang; 2020, Ji S; 2020; Ji W; 2020].

Let us consider four states: Susceptible; Carrier; Infected; and Removed for the mathematical SCIR modeling [Allen 2008]. A fraction of individuals are likely to come in contact with carriers; subjects in the carrier state are capable of infecting members of the community. These asymptomatic carriers will either come into the infected state or coming again to the susceptible state of individuals. Individuals in the diseased state are by default also carriers. The removed state includes those in the diseased state who have improved from the disease or expired. The flow of the disease is shown in Figure 6.1.

The differential equation for the SCIR propagation model is written as

$$\frac{dS(t)}{dt} = -(P_{SC} + P_{SI} + P_{SR})S(t)I(t) \tag{6.6}$$

$$\frac{dC(t)}{dt} = (P_{SC}S(t)I(t) + P_{RC}R(t) - P_{CR}C(t) - P_{CI}C(t)) \tag{6.7}$$

$$\frac{dI(t)}{dt} = (P_{CI}C(t) + P_{SI}S(t)I(t) - P_{IR}I(t)) \tag{6.8}$$

$$\frac{dR(t)}{dt} = (P_{CR}C(t) + P_{SR}S(t)I(t) + P_{IR}I(t) - P_{RC}R(t)) \tag{6.9}$$

The differential equation governing the susceptible state, in the given time, depends on the fraction of subjects vaccinated and the susceptible subjects who return from the carrier state. Asymptomatic individuals belong to the carrier state. The death of subjects in the susceptible state due to other reasons, have to be removed. P_{SC} indicates the probability that the susceptible individual is in contact with a carrier; it is generally referred to as the internal carrier contact rate. Similarly, in the carrier state the differential equation depends on the portion of the susceptible state intermingling with the carrier state. But does not depend on those individuals reverting to the susceptible state, those exiting the carrier state by being infected and also those existing the carrier state owing to natural death. Variation in the infected class depends on the fraction of carrier individuals being infected. However, infected individuals that either recover or die due to the infection and some who experience natural death have to be excluded from the infected state individuals. P_{SI} indicates the probability that the susceptible person is infected due to spread, referred to as direct infection rate. P_{CI} indicates the probability that the asymptomatic carrier is infected; that is, the carrier infection probability. The alteration in the recovery compartment depends on the fraction of individuals vaccinated, the recovered subjects from the diseased class and those who expire due to other causes. Hence, the probability of the infected individuals, cannot reacquire the disease is the assumption made. P_{IR} indicates the probability that the infected person is recovered is termed acquired immunity rate. P_{CR} indicates the probability that the carrier has recovered directly; it refers to the immunity rate.

$$\frac{dS}{dt} = (1 - p)v - \beta CS + \gamma_1 C - vS \qquad (6.10)$$

$$\frac{dC}{dt} = \beta CS - \gamma_1 C - \alpha C - vC \qquad (6.11)$$

$$\frac{dI}{dt} = \alpha C - \gamma_2 C - \mu_1 I - vI \qquad (6.12)$$

Hence the final equations are (6.4), (6.5) and (6.6). Where v is the proportion vaccinated, α is the infection rate of carriers, β is the transmission rate, γ_1 is the grade of the carriers compartment subjects who return to the susceptible compartment, $\gamma2$ depicts the infected recovery grade, $\mu 1$ is grade of death due to other causes, and $\mu 2$ is grade of death due to contagious disease. The differential equation governing the susceptible class, is given by the fraction of people vaccinated, $(1- p)$ v. The reproduction number denotes the count of ancillary infections caused by the mean of contagious individuals. The R0 of the model is obtained using the van den Driessche and Watmough algorithm, (2002), paper. The parameter x is used to depict all compartments so

$$x = \left(\frac{dS}{dt}, \frac{dC}{dt}, \frac{dI}{dt} \right)^T \qquad (6.13)$$

Then $Fi (x)$ represent the grade at which new contagious diseases appear, while $V_i^+(x)$ and $V_i^-(x)s$ are the grades where subjects enter and leave every compartment. The other parameters are defined such that $F = \left[\frac{\partial F_i}{\partial x_j}(x_0) \right]$ and $V = \left[\frac{\partial V_i}{\partial x_j}(x_0) \right]$ with $1 \le i, j \le m$; here m depicts the count of classes in which subjects suffer from the contagious disease. The reproduction number is then defined as

$$R_0 = \rho(FV^{-1}) \qquad (6.14)$$

here ρ (*A*) depicts the highest eigen value of matrix *A*. Solving the equation gives the solution as

$$R0 = \beta/\gamma_1 + \alpha + \nu \qquad (6.15)$$

The reproduction rate R0, is a significant metric for measuring the spread of COVID-19. R0 is described as the mean number of subjects affected over the COVID-19 infection period, in completely susceptible subjects. The most important solutions for the model are taking the inequality S(0) R0 > 1, then the count of affected population will swiftly decrease. Hence, no contagious spread happens during the pandemic. If S(0) R0 < 1, then a pandemic will occur even if there are very few infected among the population. The size of the pandemic will not rely on the preliminary number of infected subjects, but on the initial portion of suscep-tibles, S(0), and on R0. Several steps have to be taken to avoid pandemics by reducing the initial fraction of susceptibles to S(0) < γ_1+α +ν / β.The first measure would be to vaccinate the population to prevent the pandemic, but vaccines have not been invented as of this writing. Another way to achieve the condition S(0) < γ_1+α +ν / β, and eradicate the pandemic, is diminishing the transmissibility rate β by quarantining affected individuals. Further metrics include increasingthe recovery rate γ by speedy alternative treatment of corona-affected subjects. However, the perfect treatment has not yet been developed. Another way would be reducing carriers by sanitising efficiently. Sanitising can be done effectively using drones [Cheshmehzangi 2020a; Kummitha 2020a].

Using drones is highly commendable for their accessibility and usefulness in fogging disinfectant on buildings; it is highly difficult to perform this activity manually. The sanitisation drone uses autopilot technology, an innovative flight controller system, and a fuel-effective motor that allows the drone to be deployed for 12 hours a day. The drone has the capability to cover 20 km a day. The flight duration is 42–46 minutes, with payload capacity of 13–23 litres. They reach maximum ceiling height of 400 to 460 feet. They are capable of disinfecting up to 99% of tall buildings across India. Spraying disinfectant in public areas will curb surface spread to a great degree. Drone-based sanitising is shown Figure 6.2. Research based on studies and data obtained from several sanitization operations across the country has indicated a sudden stagnation or dip in the number if cases in the city.

Garuda Aerospace has brought a Corona-Killer Automated Disinfecting Unmanned Aerial Vehicle (UAV) that helps in sanitization of common public property, hospitals and tall buildings. These drones are used to spray disinfectants on buildings up to 450 feet. The most crucial Factor in using the drone is that the distance it can cover in a day is 20 km; a human can cover only four to five km. 300 drones can cover and disinfect 6000 linear km in a day. Drone-based solutions are meant to replace human health workers in sanitation activities and protect them from infection. The drones will do the same job and cover a lot more distance. Every day from 6 am to 6 pm, a drone works 12 hours, whereas a human being can work only 6–8 hours while carrying heavy equipment. Figure 6.2 shows a drone disinfecting a city.

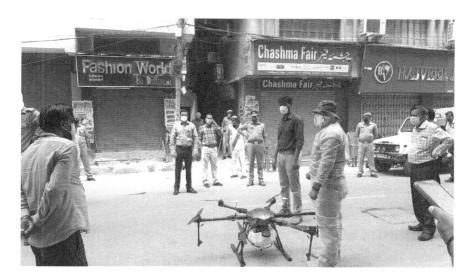

FIGURE 6.2   Varanasi being disinfected.

6.3   THERMAL IMAGING

Drones equipped with thermal sensing can help administrators recognize individuals with fibril conditions, which could indicate viral infection. Figure 6.3
shows temperatures of humans.

6.4   BROADCASTING INFORMATION

These robots can also announce messages to further localities than conventional
audio systems, while amusing the crowd.

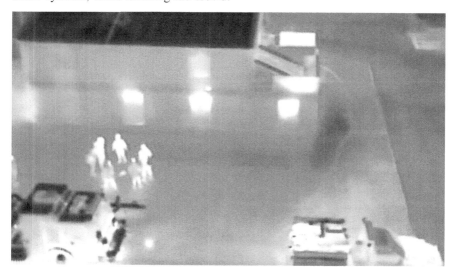

FIGURE 6.3   Thermal map of subjects during drone surveillance.

6.5   DELIVERY OF ESSENTIALS

During COVID-19, due to lockdown and quarantine, goods are delivered without human contact, but with UV sterilisation. The drones are properly sterilised and free from infection. Hence, they can be used easily to deliver essential items, like medicine and food.

6.6   PATROLLING

Drones can also be used to watch areas, and monitor gatherings and traffic jam more efficiently. Individuals not wearing masks or practicing precautions can be identified.

6.7   DISINFECTION

Spraying chemicals in hotspots kills the virus on surfaces.

6.8   RESULTS AND DISCUSSION

Disinfection was carried out in Varanasi and its effects were studied in the location. Table 6.1 shows the area covered by drones, the chemical sprayed in litres in each location and battery cycles charged to run the drones. Almost all main locations

TABLE 6.1

Hot zones in Varanasi where drone operations were carried out

Zone	Location	Area Coverage	Chemicals Used	Battery Cycle (Sorti)
1	Madhanpuraand its areas	53.22	7	10
2	Murugayyatollaand its areas	29.46	3	5
3	Pitarkundaand its areas	29.63	5	10
4	Dhanialpurand its areas	43.1	5	8
5	Shivpurand itsareas (Hospital)	58.9	4	10
6	Shivpurgarden areas	3.46	1.5	4
7	Parmanandpurand its areas	40.3	4	6
8	VikasbhavanKajori	71.5	6	10
9	BhimNagar park	73.1	6	10
10	Gangapur-registryoffice	58.1	6	8
11	GangapurMarket	5.61	1.5	2
12	Madhanpura–2rd time	23.9	5	6
13	SapthSagarMandi	58	5.5	7
14	Patrakarpuram	64.5	5.5	10
15	Municipal Corporation	67.7	10	16
16	Police Line	73	14	18
Total		**753.48**	**89**	**140**

were covered. The table shows that the drone covered 753.4 sq meters, nine litres of disinfectant were used and 140 battery cycles were used to sanitize Varanasi.

The drone used for disinfection was filled with sodium hypochlorite [NaOCl], the chemical solution recommended by WHO. The drone is standardised and conventionally prepared to fly. The drone's movements are controlled by the proficient pilots with a remote control device, which squirts the chemical solution through four nozzles. The flight lasts for approximately 15 to 20 minutes. Once the chemicals are sprayed, the drones are called back to refill the sanitizer and swap the battery pack. Once the designated area is complete, the next area is identified and spraying is resumed. The trajectory and area covered by the drone are controlled by the pilot with a handheld device. GIS maps on the back end are available in the handheld device and all movements are controlled by remote. GPS and GSM-based wireless cameras are used for monitoring the complete drone operation and control.

In this work, drone operations are centrally monitored from the Kashi Integrated Command and Control Centre, now converted to COVID-19 War Room. Figure 6.4 below shows the map of distances covered by drones in the hot spot areas.

The city's statistics were studied before and after the sanitising operation was performed. Figure 6.5 shows the average individuals in susceptible, carrier and

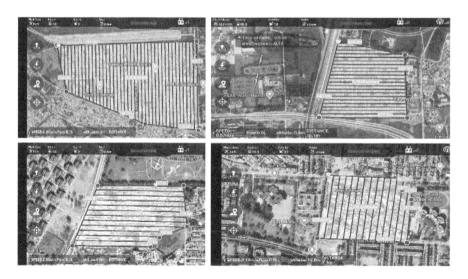

FIGURE 6.4 The sample areas covered by drones during the sanitiising operation.

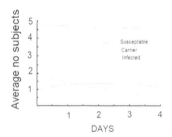

FIGURE 6.5 Average no of individuals in different class before sanitising.

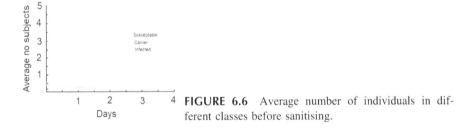

FIGURE 6.6 Average number of individuals in different classes before sanitising.

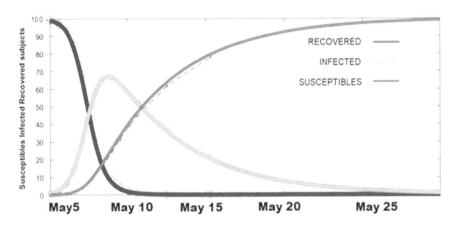

FIGURE 6.7 SIR solutions behavior in continuous time of disease outbreak.

infectious states in Varanasi before sanitising. The graph shows that the mean of cases were two before sanitising operations. After the sanitising operation was performed, the average case came down. Figure 6.6 depicts average individuals in susceptible, carrier and infectious states in Varanasi after sanitising. Microbial tests were carried out before and after sanitising. After sanitising 97.02% microorganisms on the surface was removed.

The solution of the differential equations (6.2), (6.3) and (6.4) are found by numerical analysis using python. The output graph is shown in Figure 6.7. The solution for the equation gives $\beta = 0.1$ and $\gamma = 0.7$. Ro for the area is found to be 0.1 since it less than 1. Figure 6.7 shows that the outbreak has not occured in the region. When the transmission rate is small, not everybody gets sick.

To curb the situation, the condition $S(0) < \gamma / \beta$ must be satisfied, thus reducing the possibility of infection by increasing the immunity of the community by vaccination and reduce the chance of susceptible community for catching the infection. The transmissibility parameter β can be minimized by keeping the diseased subjects away, by following measures like social distancing, performing frequent cleanising and decontamination. The recovery rate γ can be inflated by treatment of affected subjects in isolation.

Since vaccines have not yet been developed, we can combat the disease by consuming alternate medicines to increase immunity. This can reduce the susceptible S(0) < γ /β. Other measures of mitigation are implementing social distancing measures, properly cleansing surfaces and decontaminating gathering places. In this work, it is recommended that drone-based monitoring and disinfection of hotspots be carried out until a vaccine emerges. This helps to eliminate the surface spread of the virus. Statistical analysis of hotspots indicate a fall in the number of infected people in areas where drone-based implementation was carried out.

Hence it is found that, until preventive vaccination and proper drugs are available for curing the COVID-19, sanitizing is the best control measure. Sanitizing using drones was effective in monitoring and reducing infectious carrier cases.

6.9   CONCLUSION

Using a mathematical model, it was proven that control measures to prevent the spread of corono virus is to coronovirus reduce the reproduction number R0 of the model. The spread of virus could be reduced by vaccinating, increasing the immunity of the population, social distancing, finding proper drugs and sanitizing. In the case study, it was found that drone-based sanitizing was effective in containing the spread of the disease.

REFERENCES

Allen, E. J. (2009). Derivation of stochastic partial differential equations for size-and age-structured populations. *Journal of Biological Dynamics*, 3(1), 73–86.

Allen, E. J., Allen, L. J., Arciniega, A., & Greenwood, P. E. (2008). Construction of equivalent stochastic differential equation models. *Stochastic Analysis and Applications*, 26(2), 274–297.

Arif, M. S., Raza, A., Rafiq, M., Bibi, M., Fayyaz, R., Naz, M., & Javed, U. (2019). A reliable stochastic numerical analysis for typhoid fever incorporating with protection against infection. *Computers Materials and Continua*, 59(3), 787–804.

Ayittey, F. K., Dzuvor, C., Ayittey, M. K., Chiwero, N. B., & Habib, A. (2020). Updates on Wuhan 2019 novel coronavirus epidemic. *Journal of Medical Virology*, 92(4), 403.

Azamfirei, R. (2020). The 2019 novel coronavirus: a crown jewel of pandemics? *The Journal of Critical Care Medicine*, 6(1), 3–4.

Bannister, F., & Connolly, R. (2020). The future ain't what it used to be: Forecasting the impact of ICT on the public sphere. *Government Information Quarterly*, 37(1), 101410.

Bayram, M., Partal, T., & Buyukoz, G. O. (2018). Numerical methods for simulation of stochastic differential equations. *Advances in Difference Equations*, 2018(1), 1–10.

Benvenuto, D., Giovanetti, M., Ciccozzi, A., Spoto, S., Angeletti, S., & Ciccozzi, M. (2020). The 2019-new coronavirus epidemic: evidence for virus evolution. *Journal of Medical Virology*, 92(4), 455–459.

Bloom, G., MacGregor, H., McKenzie, A., & Sokpo, E. (2015). Strengthening health systems for resilience.

Calvo, R. A., Deterding, S., & Ryan, R. M. (2020). Health surveillance during COVID-19 pandemic.

Carinci, F. (2020). COVID-19-19: preparedness, decentralisation, and the hunt for patient zero.

Cavallo, L., Marcianò, A., Cicciù, M., & Oteri, G. (2020). 3D printing beyond dentistry during COVID-19 19 epidemic: A technical note for producing connectors to breathing devices. *Prosthesis*, 2(2), 46–52.

Chen, P., Chen, E., Chen, L., Zhou, X. J., & Liu, R. (2019). Detecting early-warning signals of influenza outbreak based on dynamic network marker. *Journal of Cellular and Molecular Medicine*, 23(1), 395–404.

Cheshmehzangi, A. (2020a). 10 adaptive measures for public places to face the COVID-19 19 pandemic outbreak. *City & Society*, 32(2), 12335–12345.

Cheshmehzangi, A. (2020b). How Cities Cope in Outbreak Events?. In *The City in Need* (pp. 17–39). Springer, Singapore.

Cohen, J., & Kupferschmidt, K. (2020). Strategies shift as coronavirus pandemic looms.

Colson, P., & Raoult, D. (2016). Fighting viruses with antibiotics: an overlooked path. *International Journal of Antimicrobial Agents*, 48(4), 349.

Ekanayake, A. J., & Allen, L. J. (2010). Comparison of Markov chain and stochastic differential equation population models under higher-order moment closure approximations. *Stochastic Analysis and Applications*, 28(6), 907–927.

Fiorillo, L., Cervino, G., Matarese, M., D'Amico, C., Surace, G., Paduano, V., & Laudicella, R. (2020). COVID-19Surface Persistence: A Recent Data Summary and Its Importance for Medical and Dental Settings. *International Journal of Environmental Research and Public Health*, 17(9), 3132.

Foster, K. A., Christian, D., & Matthew, K. A. (2020). Updates on Wuhan 2019 Novel Coronavirus Epidemic. *Journal of Medical Virology*, 92(4), 403–407.

GEN (2020). BGI's coronavirus response?: Building a lab in Wuhan, China. *Geneticngineering & Biotechnology News*, 40(3), 10–11.

Hansen, S., Faye, O., Sanabani, S. S., Faye, M., Böhlken-Fascher, S., Faye, O., & Abd El Wahed, A. (2018). Combination random isothermal amplification and nanopore sequencing for rapid identification of the causative agent of an outbreak. *Journal of Clinical Virology*, 106, 23–27.

Huang, J., Cheng, A., Lin, S., Zhu, Y., & Chen, G. (2020). Individualized prediction nomograms for disease progression in mild COVID-19-19. *Journal of Medical Virology*, 92(10), 2074–2080.

Ji, W., Wang, W., Zhao, X., Zai, J., & Li, X. (2020). Cross-species transmission of the newly identified coronavirus 2019-n CoV. *Journal of Medical Virology*, 92(4), 433–440.

Ji, S., Bai, Q., Wu, X., Zhang, D. W., Wang, S., Shen, J. L., & Fei, G. H. (2020). Unique synergistic antiviral effects of Shufeng Jiedu Capsule and oseltamivir in influenza A viral-induced acute exacerbation of chronic obstructive pulmonary disease. *Biomedicine & Pharmacotherapy*, 121, 109652.

Khan, S., Siddique, R., Ali, A., Xue, M., & Nabi, G. (2020). Novel coronavirus, poor quarantine, and the risk of pandemic. *Journal of Hospital Infection*, 104(4), 449–450.

Kharpal, A. (2020). Use of surveillance to fight coronavirus raises concerns about government power after pandemic ends. *CNBC*. Retrieved: 04-01-2020.

Kummitha, R. K. R. (2020a). Why distance matters: The relatedness between technology development and its appropriation in smart cities. *Technological Forecasting and Social Change*, 157, 120087.

Kummitha, R. K. R. (2020b). Smart technologies for fighting pandemics: The techno-and human-driven approaches in controlling the virus transmission. *Government Information Quarterly*, 37(3), 101481–101492.

Lam, T. T. Y., Jia, N., Zhang, Y. W., Shum, M. H. H., Jiang, J. F., Zhu, H. C., & Li, W. J. (2020). Identifying SARS-CoV-2-related coronaviruses in Malayan pangolins. *Nature*, 583(7815), 282–285.

Lee, Y. J., & Lee, C. (2016). Ivermectin inhibits porcine reproductive and respiratory syndrome virus in cultured porcine alveolar macrophages. *Archives of Virology*, 161(2), 257–268.

Li, C., & Xu, B. H. (2020). The viral, epidemiologic, clinical characteristics and potential therapy options for COVID-19-19: a review. *European Review for Medical and Pharmacological Sciences*, 24(8), 4576–4584.

Li, X., Zhao, X., & Sun, Y. (2020). The lockdown of Hubei province causing different transmission dynamics of the novel coronavirus (2019-ncov) in Wuhan and Beijing. *medRxiv*, 2020. Google Scholar.

Li, W., Guo, T., Wang, Y., & Chen, B. (2020). DR-SCIR public opinion propagation model with direct immunity and social reinforcement effect. *Symmetry*, 12(4), 584.

Li, Y., Chang, N., Han, Y., Zhou, M., Gao, J., Hou, Y., & Bai, G. (2017). Anti-inflammatory effects of Shufengjiedu capsule for upper respiratory infection via the ERK pathway. *Biomedicine & Pharmacotherapy*, 94, 758–766.

Li, X., Zai, J., Zhao, Q., Nie, Q., Li, Y., Foley, B. T., & Chaillon, A. (2020). Evolutionary history, potential intermediate animal host, and cross-species analyses of SARS-CoV-2. *Journal of Medical Virology*, 92(6), 602–611.

Liu, Z., Xiao, X., Wei, X., Li, J., Yang, J., Tan, H., & Liu, L. (2020). Composition and divergence of coronavirus spike proteins and host ACE2 receptors predict potential intermediate hosts of SARS-CoV-2. *Journal of Medical Virology*, 92(6), 595–601.

Luo, G., & Gao, S. J. (2020). Global health concerns stirred by emerging viral infections. *Journal of Medical Virology*, 92(4), 399–400.

Malik, Y. S., Sircar, S., Bhat, S., Sharun, K., Dhama, K., Dadar, M., & Chaicumpa, W. (2020). Emerging novel coronavirus (2019-nCoV)—current scenario, evolutionary perspective based on genome analysis and recent developments. *Veterinary Quarterly*, 40(1), 68–76.

McCluskey, C. C. (2010). Complete global stability for an SIR epidemic model with delay—distributed or discrete. *Nonlinear Analysis: Real World Applications*, 11(1), 55–59.

Mollison, D., & Denis, M. (Eds.). (1995). *Epidemic models: their structure and relation to data* (Vol. 5). Cambridge University Press.

Murdoch, D. R., & French, N. P. (2020). COVID-19-19: another infectious disease emerging at the animal-human interface. *The New Zealand Medical Journal (Online)*, 133(1510), 12–15.

Power, B. (2020). The coronavirus is expanding the surveillance state. How will this play out? *Washington Post: Analysis*. Retrieved: 04-01-2020.

Raza, A., Arif, M. S., & Rafiq, M. (2019). A reliable numerical analysis for stochastic dengue epidemic model with incubation period of virus. *Advances in Difference Equations*, 2019(1), 32.

Rodriguez-Morales, A. J., Bonilla-Aldana, D. K., Tiwari, R., Sah, R., Rabaan, A. A., & Dhama, K. (2020). COVID-19-19, an emerging coronavirus infection: current scenario and recent developments-an overview. *Journal of Pure and Applied Microbiology*, 14, 6150.

Romantsov, M. G., & Golofeevskiĭ, S. V. (2010). Cycloferon efficacy in the treatment of acute respiratory tract viral infection and influenza during the morbidity outbreak in 2009-2010. *Antibiotiki i Khimioterapiia= Antibiotics and Chemotherapy [sic]*, 55(1-2), 30–35.

Salata, C., Calistri, A., Parolin, C., & Palu, G. (2019). Coronaviruses: a paradigm of new emerging zoonotic diseases. *Pathogens and Disease*, 77(9), ftaa006.

Sari, E. R., & Fajar, R. (2019). Stability analysis of SCIR-SI compartmental model for meningococcal meningitis disease between two regions. *MJS*, *38*(2), 79–97.

Schwerdtle, P. M., De Clerck, V., & Plummer, V. (2017). Experiences of Ebola survivors: causes of distress and sources of resilience. *Prehospital and Disaster Medicine*, 32(3), 234.

Suroyo, G., & Allard, T. (2020). Indonesia warns of escalating coronavirus cases, adds restrictions on foreign travellers. Reuters. Retrieved from: https://www.reuters.com/article/health-coronavirus-indonesia-travel-int/indonesia-warns-of-escalating-coronavirus-cases-adds-restrictions-on-foreign-travellers-idUSKBN2141FL.

Tahir, R. F. (2020). RS Rujukan Corona di Sultra Kekurangan APD, Pakai Jas Hujan. Tempo. Retrieved from: https://nasional.tempo. co/read/1321045/rs-rujukan-corona-di-sultra-kekurangan-apd-pakai-jas-hujan.

Thompson-Dyck, K., Mayer, B., Anderson, K. F., & Galaskiewicz, J. (2016). Bringing people back in: crisis planning and response embedded in social contexts. In *Urban Resilience* (pp. 279–293). Springer, Cham.

Wang, P., Lu, J., Jin, Y., Zhu, M., Wang, L., & Chen, S. (2020). Epidemiological characteristics of 1212 COVID-19patients in Henan, China. *medRxiv*, 148, e130–137.

Watts, C. H., Vallance, P., & Whitty, C. J. (2020). Coronavirus: global solutions to prevent a pandemic. *Nature*, 578(7795), 363-363.

Winter, G. (2020). COVID-19and emergency planning. *British Journal of Community Nursing*, 25(4), 184–186.

Wood, C. (2020). Infections without borders: a new coronavirus in Wuhan, China. *British Journal of Nursing*, 29(3), 166–167.

Yang, W. (2017). *Early Warning for Infectious Disease Outbreak: Theory and Practice*. Academic Press.

Yang, Y., Shang, W., & Rao, X. (2020b). Facing the COVID-19-19 outbreak: what should we know and what could we do?. *Journal of Medical Virology*, 92(6), 536–537.

Yang, Y., Peng, F., Wang, R., Guan, K., Jiang, T., Xu, G.,... & Chang, C. (2020a). The deadly coronaviruses: the 2003 SARS pandemic and the 2020 novel coronavirus epidemic in China. *Journal of Autoimmunity*, 109, 102434–102441.

Yuan, Y., & Allen, L. J. (2011). Stochastic models for virus and immune system dynamics. *Mathematical Biosciences*, 234(2), 84–94.

Zhang, S., Tian, J., Liu, Q. L., Zhou, H. Y., He, F. R., & Ma, X. (2011). Reliability and validity of SF-12 among floating population. *Chinese Journal of Public Health*, 27(2), 226–227.

Zhou, F., Yu, T., Du, R., Fan, G., Liu, Y., Liu, Z.,... & Guan, L. (2020). Clinical course and risk factors for mortality of adult inpatients with COVID-19in Wuhan, China: a retrospective cohort study. *The lancet*, 395(10229), 1054–1062.

Zhu, S., Guo, X., Geary, K., & Zhang, D. (2020). Emerging Therapeutic Strategies for COVID-19patients. *Discoveries*, 8(1), e105.

7 ANFIS Algorithm-based Modeling and Forecasting of the COVID-19 Epidemic: A Case Study in Tamil Nadu, India

M. Vijayakarthick[1*], E. Sivaraman[2],
S. Meyyappan[1], and N. Vinoth[1]

[1]Department of Instrumentation Engineering, MIT Campus, Anna University, Chennai, India
[2]Department of Electronics and Communication Engineering, GCE, Tirunelveli, India
[*]Corresponding author E-mail id: vijayakarthick@yahoo.co.in

7.1 INTRODUCTION

The novel Coronavirus was identified by Chinese authorities on 7 January 2020 and temporarily named "COVID-19". Coronaviruses are a large group of viruses that cause sickness varying from the ordinary cold to more severe diseases. This is a new strain that has never before been recognized in human beings (Organization WH 2019). On 11 February 2020, this new virus was subsequently named COVID-19 by the World Health Organization (WHO) (Organization WH 2019). Based on the levels of spread and severity, on 11 March 2020, WHO made the observation that COVID-19 had the potential to be regarded as a pandemic (Organization WH 2020). The COVID-19 virus infects people of all age groups. The elderly and those who are being treated for underlying medical conditions are at a high risk of becoming prey to COVID-19.

From the first to the second week of June 2020, nearly 100,000 new cases were counted every day. Nearly 75% of reported cases emerged from ten countries, typically in United States of America and South Asia (Organization WH 2020). As of 24 September 2020, this outbreak had infected around 32 million people globally,

111

with 973,987 fatalities. In the first month of the outbreak, under 10,000 cases were reported to WHO. For the most recent month (August 2020), approximately 8 million cases have been reported (Organization WH 2020).

In India, the first case of COVID-19 infection was recorded on 30 January 2020 (Organization WH 2020). The Indian government took necessary steps against COVID-19, such as screening air travelers in both domestic and international airports, and shutting down factories, educational institutions and various public and private sector organizations during the first week of March 2020. In addition to that, the Government of India forced a nationwide lockdown for 21 days, in effect from 25 March until May 31 2020 (India Ministry of Home Affairs 2020). As of the end of May, 182,143 positive cases and 5,164 deaths were reported officially across the country (Organization WH 2020). Longer periods of lockdown could limit the spread of COVID-19, but after lifting lockdown orders in India on 01 June 2020, the infection rate rapidly increased. According to the government of India's official report on 24 September 2020, there were 5,732,518 COVID-19 cases in India, including 91,149 deaths and 4,674,987 recoveries (Government of India 2020).

The state of Tamil Nadu, India, witnessed its first COVID-19 case on 7 March 2020. According to a government report of 24 September 2020, 563,691 people had tested positive for COVID-19, which included 9,076 deaths and 508,210 recoveries (Health & Family Welfare Department 2020). Many progressive steps are being taken by the state government to control the transmission of the epidemic. These include lockdown, social distancing and other preventive measures, along with increasing the number of tests to identify positive cases.

The mathematical model for COVID-19 is used to determine how virological transmission takes place among people in crowded places. This model can then be used to predict pandemic situations and recommend effective control and interception methods (Cao et al. 2020). In many research articles, mathematical models are suggested to explain the dynamics of the COVID-19 epidemic (Roosa et al. 2020; Kucharski et al. 2020).

7.2   COMPUTATIONAL METHODS

Ndairou et al. (2020) suggested a mathematical model for the transmission of COVID-19, highlighting the transmissibility of super-spreading individuals. They studied the consistency of the disease in terms of the reproduction rate, and evaluated the sensitivity of the model with respect to its parameter variations. The numerical simulations illustrate the suitability of the suggested COVID-19 model for the epidemic that occurred in Wuhan province, China.

Zeb et al. (2020) presented a mathematical model of continuously varying behavior of COVID-19 infection by adding a separation class. Also they discussed positivity of the model in their work. In the suggested model, the Non-Standard Finite Difference (NSFD) scheme and Runge-Kutta fourth order (RK-4) method are used for numerical studies; simulation results are provided based on the study.

Shastri et al. (2020) developed several deep-learning algorithms for COVID-19 cases, making a comparative study of India and the United States. Here, both active and fatal cases of COVID-19 were taken into consideration for model development.

Moreover, the authors suggested Stacked LSTM, Bi-directional LSTM and Convolutional LSTM for predicting COVID-19 cases a month in advance. The trend of forecasted COVID-19 cases was analyzed and graphically represented. The Graphical representation of the forecasted trend of COVID-19 cases would be helpful for policy makers to control the death and infection rates.

Kuhl (2020) illustrated how data-driven modeling can incorporate classical epidemiology modelling and machine learning to deduce critical disease parameters in real time from reported case data. This will enable more accurate predictions. Also, the authors provided guiding principles for robust mathematical models to realize and handle the epidemic crisis.

Zhong et al. (2020) narrated an early forecast of the COVID-19 outbreak in China based on a simple mathematical model and limited epidemiological data. The model predicts that the cumulative number of COVID-19 cases may reach 76,000 to 230,000, with the peak of active cases falling between 22,000 and 74,000 by the end of February or the first week of March. After that, there may be a steady decrease in the number of active cases until first week of May to late June, as the COVID-19 outbreak will fade out during that period. The impact of the epidemic may be reduced by taking strong precautionary measures, thereby lowering the cumulative infected cases by 40%–49%. They also projected that the development of medical care could decrease transmission by one-half and efficiently cut down the duration of COVID-19.

The primary objective of this work is to develop a mathematical epidemic model for COVID-19 to estimate different conditions, such as the number of affected cases, death toll and the eventual requirement of hospital beds. The organization of this chapter is as follows; section 1 deals with introduction to COVID-19 and significance of this work. The ANFIS based predictive models for COVID-19 are depicted in section 2. Section 3 presents the outcome of predicted model analysis of the outbreak and finally the chapter is concluded in section 4.

7.3   MATHEMATICAL MODELING OF COVID-19 PANDEMIC

Since the contagion and death rates of COVID-19 increase sharply in India, it is necessary to develop a healthy model for estimating the transmission of COVID-19, so as to take both precautionary and preventive measures. Many Indian government organizations, such as the Indian Council of Medical Research (ICMR) and the Department of Science and Technology (DST), have already started to carry out research on COVID-19 to monitor the future transmission of infection, thereby helping the government to take decisions relating to the health care system (Department of Science and Technology 2020).

In Tamil Nadu, a statewide lockdown was declared on 23 March 2020 and was extended until 30 June 2020. Considering the economy of the state, the lockdown cannot go on for an indefinite period, whereas lifting the lockdown would result in a huge epidemic transmission rate. At this juncture, a mathematical model is to be developed to predict the future transmission of COVID-19 and its consequences. In this chapter, dynamic mathematical models using ANFIS are developed to predict the morbidity, fatality and active case rates of COVID-19 in the state of Tamil Nadu, India.

7.4   ADAPTIVE NEURO FUZZY INFERENCE SYSTEM (ANFIS)

Adaptive Neuro Fuzzy Inference System (Jang, 1993, Rastegar et al. 2005, Engin et al. 2004, Jang, 1996, September, Denaï et al., 2007, Denaï et al. 2004, Shoorehdeli et al., 2006,Abdulshahed et al. 2015, Hamdan and Garibaldi 2010) makes use of a mixed-learning rule to optimize the fuzzy system parameters of the Takagi-Sugeno (TS) system. The output of each rule is a linear combination of input variables; an invariable term and the weighted average of each rule's output provides the primary output. The basic ANFIS structure (refer to Figure 7.1) includes two inputs (x and y) and one output (z). The rule base consists of two Takagi-Sugeno if-then rules as follows:

If x is A_1 and y is B_1 THEN $f_1 = p_1 x + q_1 y + r_1$
If x is A_2 and y is B_2 THEN $f_2 = p_2 x + q_2 y + r_2$

The node functions of the layers are expressed below:

Layer One: Every node i in this layer is a square node with a node function as

$$O_{1,i} = \mu_{A_i}(x), \ \text{for i} = 1, 2$$

$$O_{1,i} = \mu_{B_{i-2}}(y), \ \text{for i} = 1, 2$$

where x is the input to node i and A_i or B_{i-2} is a linguistic variable labeled as small or large attached to the node. In other words, $O_{1,i}$ is the membership grade of a fuzzy set A and it denotes the degree to which the given input x satisfies the quantifier A. The fuzzy set A can have any appropriate membership functions

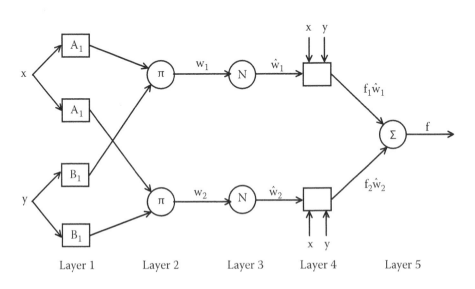

FIGURE 7.1   Basic structure of ANFIS.

such as the triangular or Gaussian functions. The chosen membership function varies in accordance with parameter changes; therefore, various forms of membership functions are available for fuzzy set A. The parameters of layer one are known as "premise parameters".

Layer Two: Layer two consists of fixed nodes; each node is labeled π, whose output is the product of all incoming signals:

$$O_{2,i} = w_i = \mu_{A_i}(x)\mu_{B_i}(y), \ i = 1, 2 \tag{7.1}$$

The output of each node denotes the firing strength of a fuzzy rule.

Layer Three: Layer three consists of fixed nodes; each node is labeled N. The ith node calculates the ratio of the firing strength at the ith instant to the sum of firing strengths of all rules:

$$O_{3,i} = w_i = w_i/(w_1 + w_2), \ i = 1, 2 \tag{7.2}$$

Outputs of this layer are called "normalized firing strengths".

Layer Four: Layer four consists of adaptive nodes; each node has a node function as

$$O_{4,i} = \overline{w_i}f_i = \overline{w_i}(p_i x + q_i y + r_i) \tag{7.3}$$

"Where $\overline{w_i}$ is a normalized firing strength from layer 3 and (p_i, q_i, r_i) is the parameter set of this node. The parameters of this layer are known as consequent parameters.

Layer Five: Layer five consists of only one fixed node labeled Σ that computes the primary output as the summation of all incoming signals:

$$\text{overall output} = O_{5,i} = \sum_i \overline{w_i}f_i = \frac{\sum_i w_i f}{\sum_i w_i} \tag{7.4}$$

7.5 FORWARD MODELING OF COVID-19 USING ANFIS

The procedure to train the ANFIS structure to represent forward dynamics of COVID-19 is called forward modeling. Forward modeling of COVID-19 uses current and past outputs to predict the current output.

The general block diagram of the forward model of process is shown in Figure 7.2. The ANFIS model is trained with 68 samples, out of which 70% is selected for training and 30% is selected for validation in order to avoid over-fitting. The parameters used for forward modeling based on ANFIS are given below:

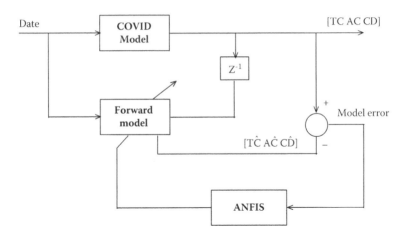

FIGURE 7.2   Forward model of COVID-19.

Input vectors	:	$[TC(k-1) \quad AC(K-1) \quad CD(K-1) \quad D(k)]$
Output vector	:	$\widehat{TC}(k) \quad \widehat{AC}(K) \quad \widehat{CD}(K)$
Sampling interval	:	1
Training	:	ANFIS
No. of clusters (c)	:	7
Membership function	:	Gbell type
Defuzzification	:	Weighted average method

Where,
   TC – Total COVID-19 affected populations
   AC – Total COVID-19 active cases
   CD – Total number of COVID-19 fatalities
   D – Date

Total infected population, active cases and death rate in the date range between 1 September 2020 to and 24 September 2020 are the inputs to the ANFIS models models. By considering these initialization parameters, the ANFIS algorithm is simulated on the Simulink platform of MATLAB software. Figures 7.3–7.5 show the membership functions for antecedent variables, which are attained by fitting the cluster projections and piece-wise exponential functions. The consequent parameters are estimated using total least square method.

In the ANFIS algorithm, the resulting part is a first-order T-S fuzzy affine model in which fuzzy rules are created for each cluster (Sivaraman and Arulselvi 2011). The resulting rule base for Total COVID-19 affected population $\widehat{TC}(k)$ is given below

1. If TC(k-1) is NB and D(K) is NB then
   $\widehat{TC}(k) = -66.79 \, TC(k-1) + 102.3 \, D(k) - 124.6$
2. If TC(k-1) is NM and D(K) is NM then
   $\widehat{TC}(k) = -6.036 \, TC(k-1) + 37.26 \, D(k) - 469.2$

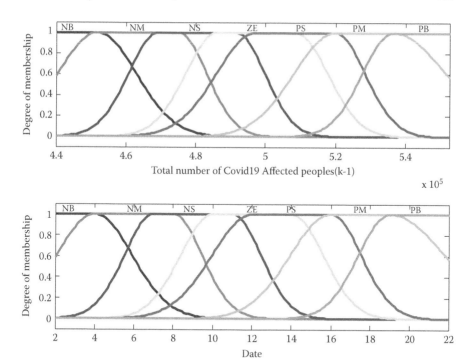

FIGURE 7.3 Membership function for total number of COVID-19 affected people in the state of Tamil Nadu, India.

3. If TC(k-1) is NS and D(K) is NS then
   $\widehat{TC}$ (k)= 10.96 TC (k-1) – 2704 D(k) – 1797
4. If TC(k-1) is ZE and D(K) is ZE then
   $\widehat{TC}$ (k)= –6.399 TC (k-1) +2706 D(k) – 72.57
5. If TC(k-1) is PS and D(K) is PS then
   $\widehat{TC}$ (k)= 5.641 TC (k-1) + 234.8 D(k) – 7.591
6. If TC(k-1) is PM and D(K) is PM then
   $\widehat{TC}$ (k)= 6.794 TC (k-1) – 4668 D(k) – 113.7
7. If TC(k-1) is PB and D(K) is PB then
   $\widehat{TC}$ (k)= –70.86 TC (k-1) + 1182 D(k) +16.24

Similarly, the resulting rule base for total COVID-19 active cases $\widehat{AC}$ (k) is given below

1. If AC(k-1) is NB and D(K) is NB then
   $\widehat{AC}$ (k)= 5.017 AC (k-1) +725.6 D(k) – 14210
2. If AC(k-1) is NM and D(K) is NM then
   $\widehat{AC}$ (k)= 21.9 AC (k-1) -344.2 D(k) – 3004
3. If AC(k-1) is NS and D(K) is NS then
   $\widehat{AC}$ (k)= -19.84 AC (k-1) + 21210 D(k) +87.35

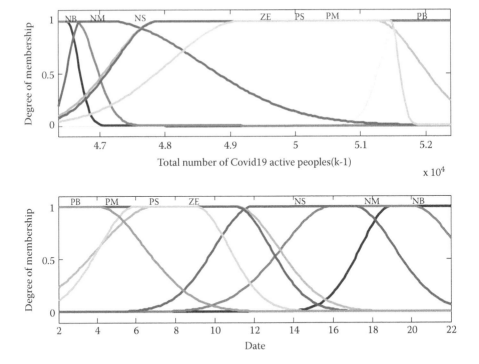

FIGURE 7.4 Membership function for total number of COVID-19 active people in the state of Tamil Nadu, India.

4. If AC(k-1) is ZE and D(K) is ZE then
   $\widehat{AC}$ (k)= –44.71 AC (k-1) +9533 D(k) – 825.8
5. If AC(k-1) is PS and D(K) is PS then
   $\widehat{AC}$ (k)= 64.92 AC (k-1) + 0.9035 D(k) – 0.8936
6. If AC(k-1) is PM and D(K) is PM then
   $\widehat{AC}$ (k)= 30.47 AC (k-1) – 3426 D(k) – 1325
7. If AC(k-1) is PB and D(K) is PB then
   $\widehat{AC}$ (k)= 21.9 AC (k-1) -344.2 D(k) – 3004

Finally, the resulting rule base for total COVID-19 deaths $\widehat{CD}$ (k) is given below

1. If CD(k-1) is NB and D(K) is NB then
   $\widehat{CD}$ (k)= –1.878 CD (k-1) – 10.9 D(k) +162.6
2. If CD(k-1) is NM and D(K) is NM then
   $\widehat{CD}$ (k)= –1.053 CD (k-1) – 3.099 D(k) +83.37
3. If CD(k-1) is NS and D(K) is NS then
   $\widehat{CD}$ (k)= –86.87 CD (k-1) + 124.3 D(k) +8.329
4. If CD(k-1) is ZE and D(K) is ZE then
   $\widehat{CD}$ (k)= 2.196 CD (k-1) +3.166 D(k) + 0.06864

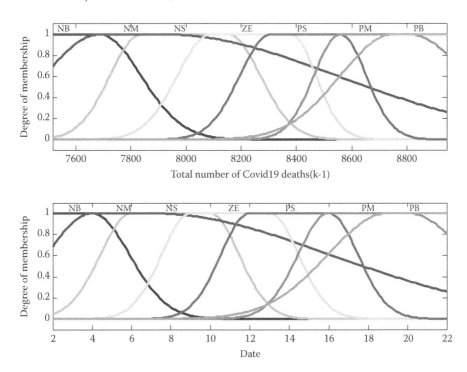

FIGURE 7.5 Membership function for total number of COVID-19 deaths in the state of Tamil Nadu, India.

5. If CD(k-1) is PS and D(K) is PS then
   $\widehat{CD}$ (k)= −0.7754 CD (k-1) + 17.25 D(k) + 0.1965
6. If CD(k-1) is PM and D(K) is PM then
   $\widehat{CD}$ (k)= −88.07 CD (k-1) + 0.04298 D(k) + 0.06933
7. If CD(k-1) is PB and D(K) is PB then
   $\widehat{CD}$ (k)= -3.18 CD (k-1) − 0.1444 D(k) − 0.0035

7.6 SIMULATION STUDY OF ANFIS MODELS FOR EPIDEMIC CASES IN THE STATE OF TAMIL NADU, INDIA

The experiments are conducted on the developed ANFIS epidemic models to reveal the competence of the proposed model-based approach by taking the COVID-19 cases in Tamil Nadu, India, into consideration.

By utilizing the total number of cases officially reported by the state government of Tamil Nadu, simulation studies are carried out using the developed ANFIS epidemic model for total number of COVID-19 affected people in the state. Figure 7.6 shows the evolution of affected cases in Tamil Nadu state, India, regarding the reported data and the predicted data attained through ANFIS epidemic model from 1 September to 24 September 2020.

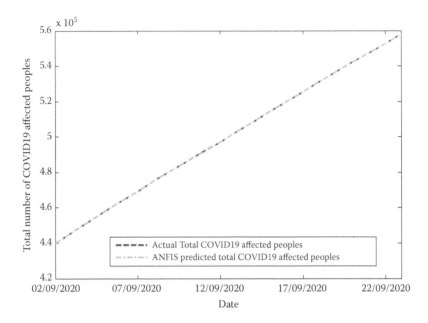

FIGURE 7.6   Evolution of total COVID-19 affected people in Tamil Nadu, India – predicted and actual data.

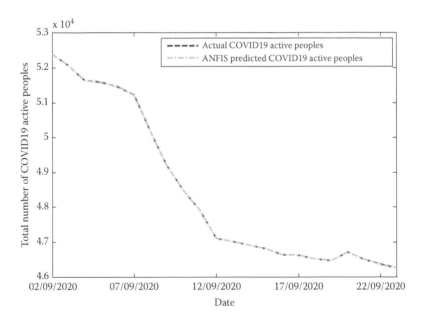

FIGURE 7.7   Evolution of total COVID-19 active people in Tamil Nadu, India - predicted and actual data.

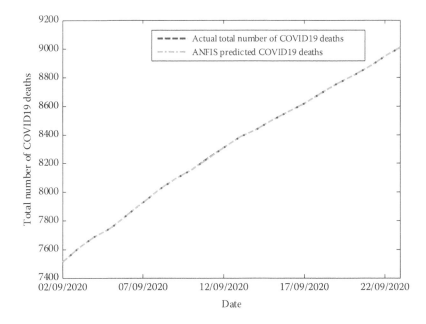

FIGURE 7.8 Evolution of total COVID-19 deaths in Tamil Nadu, India - predicted and actual data.

Likewise, two experiments were performed with proposed ANFIS model for COVID-19 active cases and COVID-19 deaths. Predicted data and reported data for both are depicted in Figure 7.7 and Figure 7.8, respectively. From the simulation results, it is noticed that the results obtained through ANFIS models fit very closely to the reported cases of the Tamil Nadu state, India, which in turn demonstrates the superiority of the proposed models in characterizing the transmission and effects of COVID-19.

7.7 THE PREDICTION OF TAMIL NADU PROVINCE EPIDEMIC

Table 7.1 presents the predicted behavior of the epidemic models such as total positive cases, total fatality rate and need for hospital beds for the months of October 2020 and November 2020.

From the Table 7.1, the following characteristics of COVID-19 are analyzed:

7.7.1 EPIDEMIC TRANSMISSION

As of September 24, 2020, 563,691 people in the Tamil Nadu state were affected with COVID-19. If not controlled, the infection rate will increase rapidly and will reach a maximum of 775,736 by the end of October 2020, and 947,522 by the end of November 2020. Table 7.1 illustrates the evolution of the weekly number of people may get affected by COVID-19 from 01 October 2020 to 30 November 2020 based on predictions made using ANFIS model. This predicted output is of great

TABLE 7.1

Prediction of parameters relating to COVID-19 for the month of October 2020 and November 2020 using ANFIS based modeling approach

Date	Total Affected Populations	Total Active Cases	Total Deaths
01/10/2020	6,03,614	47,124	9,399
15/10/2020	6,84,412	47,832	10,225
31/10/2020	7,75,736	56,350	11,162
01/11/2020	7,81,507	56,614	11,223
15/11/2020	8,61,618	60,275	12,051
30/11/2020	9,47,522	64,167	12,936

importance, as it is used to envisage the transmission of COVID-19, which in turn helps government authorities lay down control measures.

7.7.2 ACTIVE CASES

According to data reported by the state government, infected cases on 24 September 2020, around 46,249 people, are admitted to hospital. The ANFIS model forecasts quite reasonably the number of hospitalized people will be around 56,350 by the end of October 2020 and 64,167 by November 31, 2020. From the predicted data, it is clear that more beds will be urgently needed in hospitals in the state of Tamil Nadu, India.

7.7.3 FATALITY RATE

Focusing on the number of deaths, the proposed model predicted about 11,162 by the end of October 2020 and 12,936 by November 30, 2020. Thus, we strongly recommend that precautionary measures such as wearing masks, avoiding unnecessary outings and maintaining social distance should be exercised in order to fight the spread of COVID-19 in the state of Tamil Nadu.

Finally, we observe that the ANFIS epidemic models are able to predict the evolution of COVID-19 cases, which includes death rate and amount of hospitalized people, fairly well and extremely close to the actual outcome. This indicates that the proposed models using ANFIS approach can be used as decision tools to assist the authorities of the government of Tamil Nadu, India, in combating COVID-19.

7.8 CONCLUSION

In this chapter, we have presented an efficient model-based approach using ANFIS strategy for the novel SARS- CoV-2 (COVID-19) to forecast the total number of affected people, deaths rates and active cases in the state of Tamil Nadu, India, in an effort to characterize the deadly influence of the pandemic. Further, the developed models were tested in simulation with future inputs; the predicted results foresee the trend of epidemic transmission in the state of Tamil Nadu, India. The models can be used as authentic tools to control the spread of the COVID-19 pandemic.

ACKNOWLEDGMENTS

We wish to extend our heartfelt thanks to Health & Family Welfare Department, Government of Tamil Nadu and Government of India for their daily updates regarding the COVID-19 pandemic and the ease of access of this vital information as open-source data.

REFERENCES

Abdulshahed, A. M., Longstaff, A. P., & Fletcher, S. (2015). The application of ANFIS prediction models for thermal error compensation on CNC machine tools. *Applied Soft Computing*, 27, 158–168.

Cao, J., Jiang, X., & Zhao, B. (2020). Mathematical modeling and epidemic prediction of COVID-19 and its significance to epidemic prevention and control measures. *Journal of Biomedical Research & Innovation*, 1(1), 1–19.

Denaï, M. A., Palis, F., & Zeghbib, A. (2007). Modeling and control of non-linear systems using soft computing techniques. *Applied Soft Computing*, 7(3), 728–738.

Denaï, M. A., Palis, F., & Zeghbib, A. (2004, October). ANFIS based modelling and control of non-linear systems: a tutorial. In *2004 IEEE International Conference on Systems*, Man and Cybernetics (IEEE Cat. No. 04CH37583) (Vol. 4, pp. 3433–3438). IEEE.

Department of Science and Technology, Government of India, (2020). *DST initiates COVID-19 India National Supermodel for monitoring infection transmission & aid decision-making by policymakers*. URL: https://dst.gov.in/dst-initiates-COVID-19-india-national-supermodel-monitoring-infection-transmission-aid-decision#:~:text=The%20Department%20of%20Science%20and,readiness%20and%20other%20mitigation%20measures. [Accessed 24 September 2020]

Engin, S. N., Kuvulmaz, J., & Ömürlü, V. E. (2004). *Fuzzy control of an ANFIS model representing a nonlinear liquid-level system. Neural Computing & Applications*, 13(3), 202–210.

Governmentof India, (2020, September 24). *COVID-19 daily updates*. https://www.mygov.in/COVID-19/ [Accessed 24 September 2020]

Hamdan, H., & Garibaldi, J. M. (2010, July). Adaptive neuro-fuzzy inference system (ANFIS) in modelling breast cancer survival. In *International Conference on Fuzzy Systems* (pp. 1–8). IEEE.

Health & Family Welfare Department, Government of Tamil Nadu, (2020, September 24). *Daily report on Public Health measures taken for COVID-19*. https://stopcorona.tn.gov.in/wp-content/uploads/2020/09/Media-Bulletin-24.09.2020-23-Pages-English-464-KB.pdf [Accessed 24 September 2020]

India Ministry of Home Affairs, (2020, March 24) Order No. 40-3/2020-DM-I(A) URL: https://www.mha.gov.in/sites/default/files/MHAorder%20copy.pdf [Accessed 24September 2020]

Jang, J. S. (1993). ANFIS: *adaptive-network-based fuzzy inference system. IEEE Transactions on Systems, Man, and Cybernetics*, 23(3), 665–685.

Jang, J. S. (1996, September). Input selection for ANFIS learning. In *Proceedings of IEEE 5th International Fuzzy Systems* (Vol. 2, pp. 1493–1499). IEEE.

Kucharski, A. J., Russell, T. W., Diamond, C., Liu, Y., Edmunds, J., Funk, S., … & Davies, N. (2020). Early dynamics of transmission and control of COVID-19: a mathematical modelling study. *The Lancet Infectious Diseases*, 20(5): 553–558.

Kuhl, E. (2020). Data-driven modeling of COVID-19—Lessons learned. *Extreme Mechanics Letters*, 40(2020), 1–10.

Ndairou, F., Area, I., Nieto, J. J., & Torres, D. F. (2020). *Mathematical modeling of COVID-19 transmission dynamics with a case study of Wuhan* (pp. 109846). Chaos, Solitons & Fractals.

Organization WH, (2019, December 13). *Coronavirus disease (COVID-19) pandemic*. URL: https://www.euro.who.int/en/health-topics/health-emergencies/coronavirus-COVID-19/novel-coronavirus-COVID-19. [Accessed 24 September 2020]

Organization WH, (2019). *Naming the coronavirus disease (COVID-19) and the virus that causes it*. URL: https://www.who.int/emergencies/diseases/novel-coronavirus-2019/technical-guidance/naming-the-coronavirus-disease-(covid-2019)-and-the-virus-that-causes-it. [Accessed 24 September 2020]

Organization WH, (2020, March 11). *Coronavirus disease (COVID-19) situation report-51*. URL: https://www.who.int/docs/default-source/coronaviruse/situation-reports/20200311-sitrep-51-COVID-19.pdf?sfvrsn=1ba62e57_10 [Accessed 24 September 2020]

Organization WH, (2020, June 15). *Director-General's opening remarks at the media briefing onCOVID-19*. URL: https://www.who.int/dg/speeches/detail/who-director-general-s-opening-remarks-at-the-media-briefing-on-COVID-19---15-june-2020. [Accessed 24 September 2020]

Organization WH, (2020, June 24). *WHO Director-General's opening remarks at the media briefing on COVID-19*. URL: https://www.who.int/dg/speeches/detail/who-director-general-s-opening-remarks-at-the-media-briefing-on-COVID-19---24-june-2020. [Accessed 24 September 2020]

Organization WH, (2020, June 24). *Novel Coronavirus (COVID-19). India Situation Report-1*. URL: https://www.who.int/docs/default-source/wrindia/india-situation-report-1.pdf?sfvrsn=5ca2a672_0 [Accessed 24 September 2020]

Organization WH, (2020, May 31). *Novel Coronavirus (COVID-19). India Situation Report-18*. URL: https://www.who.int/docs/default-source/wrindia/situation-report/india-situation-report-18.pdf?sfvrsn=7c00a3f_2 [Accessed 24 September 2020]

Rastegar, F., Araabi, B. N., & Lucast, C. (2005, September). An evolutionary fuzzy modeling approach for ANFIS architecture. In *2005 IEEE Congress on Evolutionary Computation* (Vol. 3, pp. 2182–2189). IEEE.

Roosa, K., Lee, Y., Luo, R., Kirpich, A., Rothenberg, R., Hyman, J. M., … & Chowell, G. (2020). Real-time forecasts of the COVID-19 epidemic in China from February 5th to February 24th, 2020. *Infectious Disease Modelling*, 5, 256–263.

Shastri, S., Singh, K., Kumar, S., Kour, P., & Mansotra, V. (2020). Time series forecasting of COVID-19 using deep learning models: India-USA comparative case study. *Chaos, Solitons & Fractals*, 140, 110227.

Shoorehdeli, M. A., Teshnehlab, M., & Sedigh, A. K. (2006, June). A novel training algorithm in ANFIS structure. In *2006 American Control Conference* (pp. 6). IEEE.

Sivaraman, E., & Arulselvi, S. (2011). Modeling of an inverted pendulum based on fuzzy clustering techniques. *Expert Systems with Applications*, 38(11), 13942–13949.

Zeb, A., Alzahrani, E., Erturk, V. S., & Zaman, G. (2020). Mathematical model for coronavirus disease 2019 (COVID-19) containing isolation class. *BioMed Research International, 2020*.

Zhong, L., Mu, L., Li, J., Wang, J., Yin, Z., & Liu, D. (2020). Early prediction of the 2019 novel coronavirus outbreak in the mainland china based on simple mathematical model. *IEEE Access*, 8, 51761–51769.

8 Prediction and Analysis of SARS-CoV-2 (COVID-19) epidemic in India using LSTM Network

A. Ganesh Ram[1], S. Prabha[2], and M. Vijayakarthick[1]*

[1]Department of Instrumentation Engineering, MIT Campus, Anna University, Chennai, India

[2]Department of ECE, Hindustan Institute of Technology and Science, Chennai, India

8.1 INTRODUCTION

COVID-19 arose in Wuhan, China, and was characterised initially as a type of pneumonia. In February 2020, it was declared a global pandemic by WHO. It was called Severe Acute Respiratory Syndrome (SARS-COV-2) and caused severe sickness and death among humans. The world has struggled with infectious diseases at different times, some with incomprehensible issues. One of the earliest, the Black Death, occurred in the 14th century. In 1918, Spanish flu, which originated in France, resulted in approximately 500 million deaths globally. Asian Flu, which emerged from China in 1957, killed 1.1 million. A virus started in 1968 in Hong Kong, and Swine flu emanated from the United States in 2009. In 2003, SARS emerge from China, Ebola emerged from Zaire in 2014, Zika virus emerged from Brazil in 2015, and finally, coronavirus emerged from China in 2020 (Allam et al., 2020).

Considerable time is needed to identify various types of viruses. Improvements in technology help decrease time needed to identify viruses. It was confirmed in the recent case of COVID-19, requiring only days for identification of the disease. Recent case of Covid-19 requires less number of days for identification of disease. This updation is possible in computing scope by the development and comprehensive engagement of different technologies such as Machine learning, AI, cloud computing and big data. This technology can process and evaluate enormous

125

amounts of data from assorted sources in real time. This leads to a process for intelligent forecasting (Singh et al., 2020).

Machine learning methods have been applied for different applications in medical field for automatic diagnosis. Therefore, clinicians have believed that it plays a vital role as well as adjunct tool for medical diagnosis (Litjens et al., 2017). The advancement in this method empowers the establishment of end to end models for accomplishment of guaranteed outcome from the input data, without the demand of extraction of features manually (Punn et al., 2020).

LSTM networks have been used successfully in many fields, such as forecasting stock prices, detection of target objects in video processing, image compression and medical image segmentation (Qiu et al., 2020; Liu et al., 2019; Toderici et al., 2017; Gao et al., 2018). The COVID-19 epidemic's rapid acceleration requires proficiency in this area. Establishment of system, which will be detected automatically with the help of AI technology providing a greater number of clinical experts for all hospitals, is a difficult task owed to the minimal number of radiologists. Thus, clear, authentic and rapid AI models are very useful in overcoming the above issues and can help provide prompt aid to patients (Narin et al., 2020).

Radiologists' involvement is vital because of their abundant contributions in this area. Advancement in AI technologies for radiology help make accurate diagnoses. Further, new developments in AI technology have played an effective role in eradicating drawbacks, such as insufficient test kits, cost of the process and time delay of results. Therefore, it is essential to evolve a new AI-based prediction technique which will help investigate COVID-19 cases in the early stages without the involvement of radiologist.

In this work, an LSTM network is proposed for automatic diagnosis of COVID-19. The proposed system has an end-to-end model without considering the extraction of features; it only needs raw images to make a diagnosis.

8.2   DATA SOURCE

We have used Indian COVID-19 data available publicly. The three primary sources of the data are the Ministry of Health and Family Welfare, India (https://www.mohfw.gov.in), and COVID-19 India (https://www.covid19india.org) (MoHFW, 2020; covid19india, 2020) and Indian Council of Medical Research, Government of India, ICMR (2020) (https://www.icmr.gov.in).

8.3   CURRENT SCENARIO OF SARS-COV-2 (COVID-19) IN INDIA

The first SARS-CoV-2-positive case in India was reported in the state of Kerala on 30th January, 2020. According to the press release by the Indian Council of Medical Research (ICMR), the cumulative total samples tested up to 31st July, 2020 were **19,358,659** by 1,339 government and private laboratories in India. The ICMR reported the samples were tested in Real-Time RT PCR for COVID-19 in 684 laboratories (Govt.: 416 + Private 268), TrueNat Test for COVID-19 in 551 laboratories (Govt.: 465 + Private: 86) and CBNAAT Test for COVID-19 in 104 laboratories (Govt.: 30 + Private: 74) (ICMR, 2020). Figure 8.1 shows the

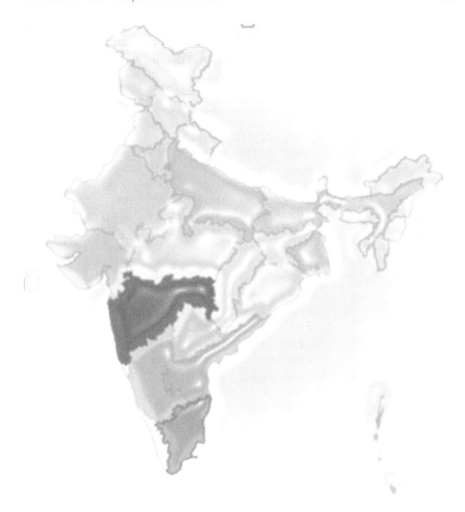

FIGURE 8.1   Geo-temporal spread of SARS-CoV-2 (COVID-19) – Total Confirmed cases in India at state level from 30th January, 2020 to 31th July, 2020.
Source: Data compiled by India in Data (https://covid19india.org), data as of 31th July, 2020.

geo-temporal spread in India from 30th January, 2020 to 31th July, 2020. Maharashtra and Tamil Nadu are the major affected states in India.

8.4   STUDY DAILY INFECTION AND DEATH RATES IN STATES

Shown in Table 8.1 are confirmed, recovered, deceased and active SARS-CoV-2 (COVID-19) cases in India, listed by state. In India, among 16,97,054 confirmed cases, 64.6% (1,095,647) recovered, 33.3% (564,856) were active cases and 2.1% (36,551) died. More than 60% of the SARS-CoV-2 (COVID-19) cases in India are in Maharashtra (24.9%), Tamil Nadu (14.5%), Andhra Pradesh (8.3%), Delhi (8%) and Karnataka (7.3%). As compared with the top five affected states, the highest

TABLE 8.1

State-by-state conformed, recovered active and death cases in India COVID-19 as of 31st July, 2020

State	Confirmed	Recovered, *%		Active, *%		Deceased, *%	
Maharashtra	4,22,118	2,56,158	(60.7%)	1,50,966	(35.8%)	14,994	(3.6%)
Tamil Nadu	2,45,859	1,83,956	(74.8%)	57,968	(23.6%)	3,935	(1.6%)
Andhra Pradesh	1,40,933	63,864	(45.3%)	75,720	(53.7%)	1,349	(1%)
Delhi	1,35,598	1,20,930	(89.2%)	10,705	(7.89%)	3,963	(2.9%)
Karnataka	1,24,115	49,788	(40.1%)	72,013	(58%)	2,314	(1.9%)
Uttar Pradesh	85,461	48,863	(57.2%)	34,968	(40.9%)	1,630	(1.9%)
West Bengal	70,188	48,374	(68.9%)	20,233	(28.8%)	1,581	(2.3%)
Telangana	62,703	45,388	(72.4%)	16,796	(26.8%)	519	(0.8%)
Gujarat	61,438	45,009	(73.3%)	13,993	(22.8%)	2,436	(4%)
Bihar	50,987	33,650	(66%)	17,039	(33.4%)	298	(0.6%)
Rajasthan	42,083	29,845	(70.9%)	11,558	(27.5%)	680	(1.6%)
Assam	40,270	30,358	(75.4%)	9,814	(24.4%)	98	(0.2%)
Haryana	34,965	28,227	(80.7%)	6,317	(18.1%)	421	(1.2%)
Odisha	31,877	20,518	(64.4%)	11,145	(35%)	214	(0.7%)
Madhya Pradesh	31,806	22,271	(70%)	8,668	(27.3%)	867	(2.7%)
Kerala	23,614	13,023	(55.1%)	10,517	(44.5%)	74	(0.3%)
Jammu and Kashmir	20,359	12,217	(60%)	7,765	(38.1%)	377	(1.9%)
Punjab	16,119	10,734	(66.6%)	4,999	(31%)	386	(2.4%)
Jharkhand	11,314	4,343	(38.4%)	6,865	(60.7%)	106	(0.9%)
Chhattisgarh	9,192	6,230	(67.8%)	2,908	(31.6%)	54	(0.6%)
Uttarakhand	7,183	4,168	(58%)	2,935	(40.9%)	80	(1.1%)
Goa	5,913	4,211	(71.2%)	1,657	(28%)	45	(0.8%)
Tripura	4,996	3,327	(66.6%)	1,648	(33%)	21	(0.4%)
Pondicherry	3,472	2,100	(60.5%)	1,323	(38.1%)	49	(1.4%)
Manipur	2,621	1,689	(64.4%)	927	(35.4%)	5	(0.2%)
Himachal Pradesh	2,564	1,459	(56.9%)	1092	(42.6%)	13	(0.5%)
Nagaland	1,693	635	(37.5%)	1,054	(62.3%)	4	(0.2%)
Arunachal Pradesh	1,591	918	(57.7%)	670	(42.1%)	3	(0.2%)
Ladakh	1,404	1,095	(78%)	302	(21.5%)	7	(0.5%)
Dadra and Nagar, Daman and Diu	1,149	725	(63.1%)	422	(36.7%)	2	(0.2%)
Chandigarh	1,051	667	(63.5%)	369	(35.1%)	15	(1.4%)
Meghalaya	823	215	(26.1%)	603	(73.3%)	5	(0.6%)
Sikkim	639	231	(36.2%)	407	(63.7%)	1	(0.2%)
Andaman and Nicobar Islands	548	214	(39.1%)	329	(60%)	5	(0.9%)
Mizoram	408	247	(60.5%)	161	(39.5%)	0	(0%)
India	**1,697,054**	**10,95,647**	**(64.6%)**	**5,64,856**	**(33.3%)**	**36,551**	**(2.2%)**

Notes:

*   *The percentages are calculated based on the total confirmed cases in each state.* Source: Data compiled by India in Data (https://api.covid19india.org/csv/latest /state_wise.csv), as of 31th July, 2020.

recovery rate of 120,930 (89.2%) occurred in Delhi for confirmed cases of 135,598. The state of Andhra Pradesh has the lowest death rate of 0.95%. The state of Tamil Nadu has the second highest recovery rate of 183,956 (74.8%) and also the second lowest death rate of 3,935 (1.6%). Only the state of Mizoram has no deaths registered till 31th July, 2020 from 408 confirmed cases.

Figure 8.1 shows a 2D combo chart for the top 16 affected SARS-CoV-2 (COVID-19) states in India. The total confirmed and total recovered cases are plotted using left side scale and total deceased cases plotted using right side scale. In the state of Gujarat, the highest percentage of death (4%) was recorded for its total confirmed cases. The second highest percentage of death (3.6%) was registered for the state of Maharashtra.

The epidemic growth of total confirmed (1,697,054), total recovered (1,095,647), total active (564,856) and total deceased (36,551) SARS-CoV-2 (COVID-19) cases in India are shown in Figure 8.2. In total confirmed cases, the recovery rate is 64.6%, the overall death rate is 2.2% and the remaining 33.3% of total active cases are admitted to hospitals. The epidemic growth of confirmed cases for the top ten states in India is shown in Figures 8.3 and 8.4.

The Table 8.2 shows the month wise percentage report for total confirmed, total recovered, total active and total deceased SARS-COV-2 (COVID-19) cases in India from January-2020 to July-2020. The percentage of total confirmed, total

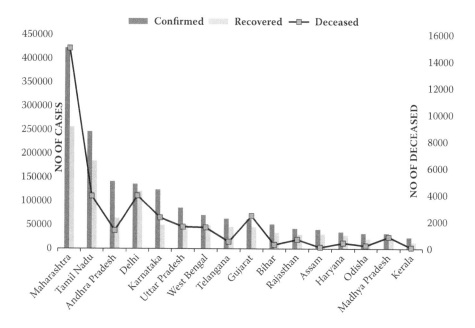

FIGURE 8.2 Graph shows the 2D combo chart of total confirmed and total recovered as plotted left side scale and total deceased as plotted right side scale for *SARS-CoV-2 (COVID-19)* cases in India.

Source: Data compiled by India in Data (https://api.covid19india.org/csv/latest/ case_time_ series.csv), data as of 31th July, 2020.

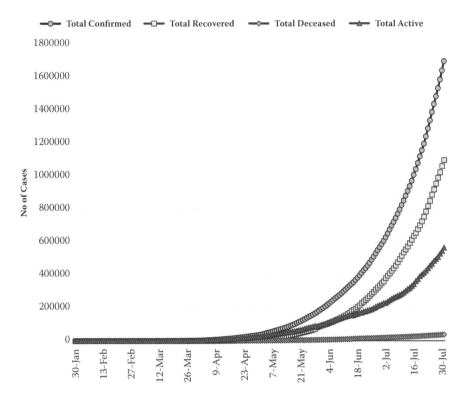

FIGURE 8.3   Graph shows the epidemic growth of total confirmed, total recovered and total deceased *SARS-CoV-2 (COVID-19)* cases in India.
Source: Data compiled by India in Data (https://api.covid19india.org/csv/latest /case_time_ series.csv), data as of 31th July, 2020.

recovered, total active and total deceased cases are calculated by using its corresponding total columns and the percentages of recovered, active and deceased cases are calculated by its total confirmed cases in its corresponding months and also listed in Table 8.2. In the month of July-2020 there are 65.5% of positive confirmed cases has registered out of 16,97,054 cases and also the highest recovery rate of 67.3% and lowest death rate of 1.72%. The month wise growth of total confirmed, total recovered, total active and total deceased cases in India as shown in Figure 8.5.

8.5   METHODS-LSTM NETWORK MODEL USING PYTHON

Python is a popular and powerful interpreted language. Python is a complete language and platform for both research and development. It is a tool to deploy and implement machine learning and deep learning, and is easy to maintain and robust. Some years ago, Python didn't have many data analysis or machine-learning libraries. Recently, Python is catching up and provides cutting-edge technology for Deep Learning (DL) or Artificial Intelligence (AI).

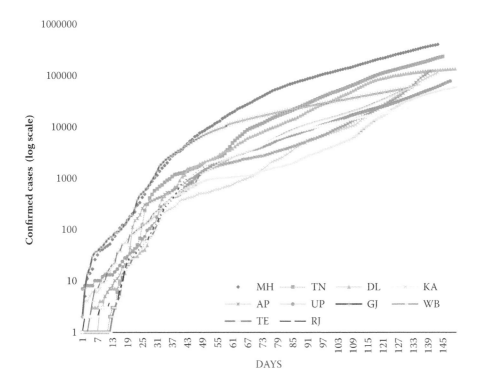

FIGURE 8.4 Graph shows the growth of total confirmed cases for top 10 states in India; the y-axis is log-scaled. The plotted states are *Maharashtra, Tamil Nadu, Delhi, Karnataka, Andhra Pradesh, Uttar Pradesh, Gujarat, West Bengal, Telangana and Rajasthan.*
Source: Data compiled by India in Data (https://api.covid19india.org/csv/latest/states.csv), data as of 31th July, 2020.

Long Short-Term Memory (LSTM) (Aroraa et al., 2020) is a Recurrent Neural Network (RNN) which contains complex computational logic. To achieve high accuracy, researchers always build large-scale LSTM networks, which are time-consuming. Instead of neurons, LSTM networks have memory blocks that are connected through layers. A block has components that make it smarter than a classical neuron and a memory for recent sequences. A block contains gates that manage the block's state and output. A block operates upon an input sequence and each gate within a block uses the sigmoid activation units to control whether they are triggered or not, making the change of state and addition of information flowing through the block conditional.

Central Idea: A memory cell (interchangeable block) which can maintain its state over time, consisting of an explicit memory (aka the cell state vector) and gating units, which regulate the information flow into and out of the memory. Cell state vector represents the memory of the LSTM (Tomar et al. 2020); it undergoes changes via forgetting of old memory (forget gate) and addition of new memory (input gate).

TABLE 8.2
Monthly total confirmed, total recovered, total active and total deceased cases in India

Date	Total Confirmed	Total Recovered	Total Active	Total Deceased	Recovered (%)	Active (%)	Deceased (%)
January-2020	1 (0%)	0 (0%)	1 (0%)	0 (0%)	0	100	0
February-2020	2 (0%)	2 (0%)	0 (0%)	0 (0%)	100	0	0
March-2020	1,632 (0.1%)	158 (0.01%)	1,427 (0.25%)	47 (0.13%)	9.68	87.4	2.88
April-2020	33,232 (1.96%)	8,899 (0.81%)	23,226 (4.11%)	1,107 (3.03%)	26.8	69.9	3.33
May-2020	1,55,781 (9.18%)	82,803 (7.56%)	68,727 (12.2%)	4,251 (11.6%)	53.2	44.1	2.73
June-2020	3,95,144 (23.3%)	2,55,977 (23.4%)	1,27,163 (22.5%)	12,004 (32.8%)	64.8	32.2	3.04
July-2020	11,11,262 (65.5%)	7,47,808 (68.3%)	3,44,312 (61%)	19,142 (52.4%)	67.3	31	1.72
Total	**16,97,054**	**10,95,647**	**5,64,856**	**36,551**	**64.6**	**33.3**	**2.15**

Memory Update: The cell state vector aggregates the two components (old memory via the forget gate and new memory via the input gate) There are three types of gates within a unit:

- **Input Gate**: Discovers which value from input should be used to modify the memory. Sigmoid function decides which values to let through; 0,1 and tanh functions give weight to the values, which are passed depending on their level of importance ranging from -1 to 1.

$$i_t = \sigma(W_i \cdot [h_{t-1}, x_t] + b_i)$$

$$\tilde{C}_t = tanh(W_c \cdot [h_{t-1}, x_t] + b_c)$$

- **Forget Gate**: Discovers what details should be discarded from the block. It is decided by the sigmoid function. It looks at the previous state (ht-1) and the content input (Xt) and outputs a number between 0 (*omit this*) and 1 (*keep this*) for each number in the cell state Ct−1.

$$f_t = \sigma(W_f \cdot [h_{t-1}, x_t] + b_f)$$

- **Output Gate:** The input and the memory of the block are used to decide the output. Sigmoid function decides which values to let through; 0,1 and tanh functions give weight to the values, which are passed depending on their level of importance ranging from-1 to 1, then multiplied with output of Sigmoid.

$$o_t = \sigma(W_o \cdot [h_{t-1}, x_t] + b_o)$$

$$h_t = o_t * tanh(c_t)$$

Each unit is like a mini-state machine where the gates of the units have weights that are learned during the training procedure.

8.6   LSTM NETWORK IMPLEMENTATION

The LSTM network implementation can be achieved to include the important libraries like panda, sklearn, keras, numpy and scipy. The state daily.csv data are imported from **api.covid19india.org/csv.** Active cases can be grouped by status, such as confirmed, recovered and deceased. The active cases are added to the DataFrame ('Active'). The total length of all grouped data are split data into X_train (85%) and X_test (15%) as input and Y_train and y_test as output. The LSTM networks model has been developed with the help of X_train, y_train and validated using x_test and y_test data.

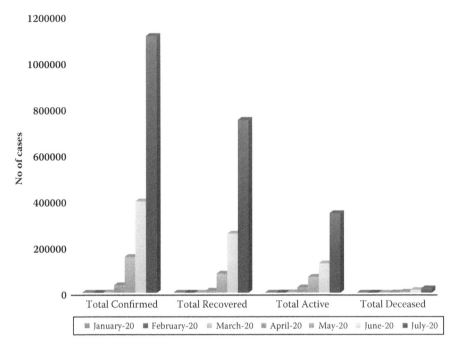

FIGURE 8.5   Graph shows the monthly growth of total confirmed, total recovered, total active and total deceased cases in India.
Source: Data compiled by India Data (https://api.covid19india.org/csv/latest/case_time_series.csv), data as of 31th July, 2020.

- The LSTM network has a visible layer with sequence inputs of 1 batch and it can be trained for 100 epochs.
- A hidden layer with 1 LSTM neurons.
- An output layer makes sequence prediction values.
- The LSTM model has add with *Dense(1)* and compile using mean square error in '*adam*' optimizer.
- The '*relu*' activation function is used for the LSTM network model.
- The LSTM model fit with X_train and y_test data with batch size of 1 and verbose=0.
- The model prediction can be performed with X_test and y_test data.
- The history of RMSE values for both train and test are held in *DateFrame()*.
- The accuracy score can be calculated with y_test and y_pred data.

Figures 8.6 and 8.7 show RMSE values for train and test data using LSTM network model for confirmed COVID-19 cases. LSTM model was used to train 85% of daily confirmed cases with data from 30th January, 2020 for 500 epochs. After completing the epochs to validate, the predicted output is compared with the remaining 15% test data as shown in Figure 8.8. An accuracy score of 70.56% was found.

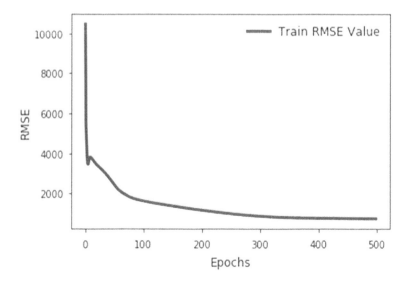

FIGURE 8.6   RMSE values during training for confirmed cases.

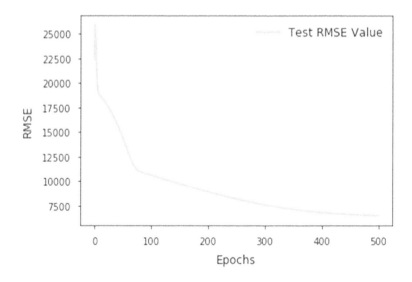

FIGURE 8.7   RMSE values during testing for confirmed cases.

Figures 8.9 and 8.10 show the RMSE values for train and test data using LSTM network model for active COVID-19 cases respectively. The LSTM model considered 90% of daily confirmed cases as X_train and active cases as y_train from 30th January, 2020 with 100 epochs. After completing the epochs to validate, the predicted active output was compared with the remaining 10% test data as shown in Figure 8.11. An accuracy score of 72.22% was found.

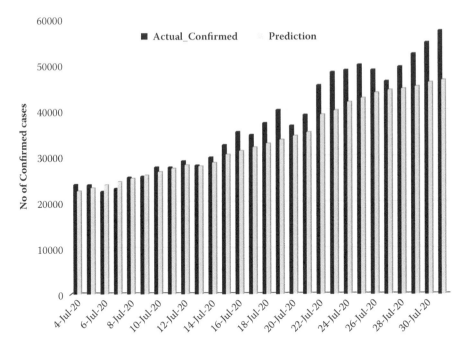

FIGURE 8.8   Daily actual confirmed cases and LSTM model prediction confirmed cases.

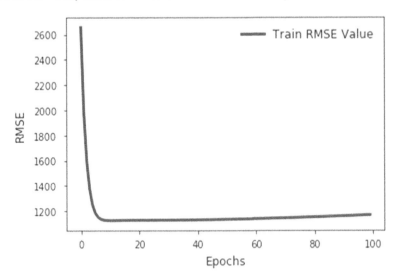

FIGURE 8.9   RMSE values during training for active case.

Figures 8.10 and 8.11 show the RMSE values for train and test data using LSTM network model for active COVID-19 cases, respectively. The LSTM model considered 90% of daily confirmed cases as X_train and active cases as y_train from 30th January, 2020 with 100 epochs. After completing the epochs to validate, the

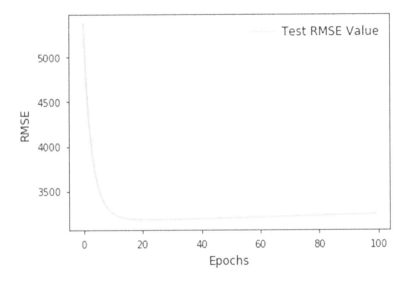

FIGURE 8.10   RMSE values during testing for active case.

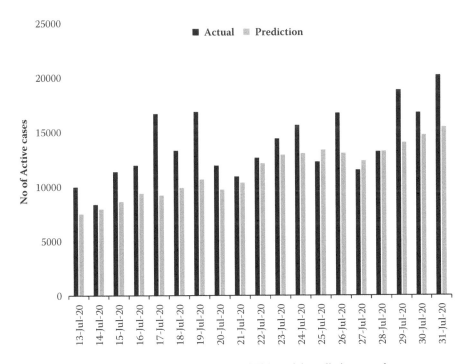

FIGURE 8.11   Daily actual active cases and LSTM model prediction actual cases.

predicted active output was compared with the remaining 10% test data as shown in Figure 8.12. An accuracy score of 72.22% was found.

Figures 8.12 and 8.13 show the RMSE values for train and test data using LSTM network model for daily deceased COVID-19 cases respectively. The LSTM model was used to train 85% of daily confirmed data as X_train and

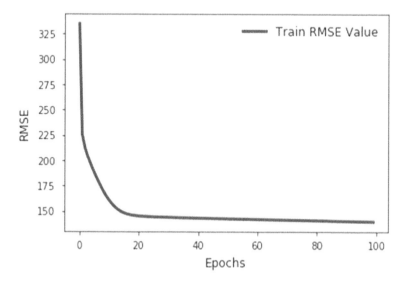

FIGURE 8.12   RMSE value during training for deceased cases.

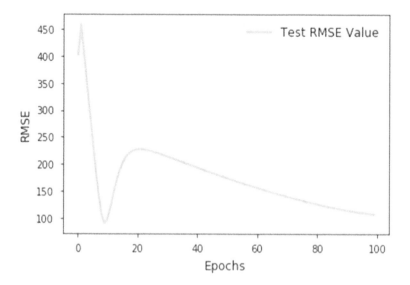

FIGURE 8.13   RMSE value during testing for deceased cases.

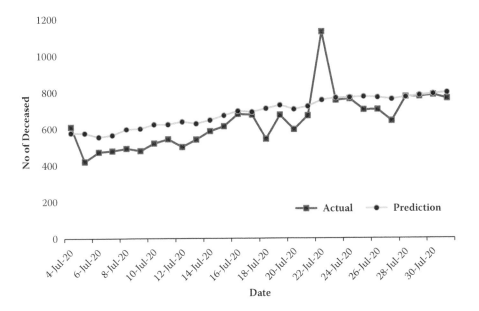

FIGURE 8.14   Daily deceased cases with LSTM model prediction deceased cases

deceased data as y_train from 30th January, 2020, with total 100 epochs. After completing the epoch to validate, the predicted deceased output data are compared with the remaining 15% test data, as shown in Figure 8.14. The accuracy score can be calculated by fitting the test data to the model output data (prediction data). The accuracy score of 70.37% was observed for daily deceased cases, daily confirmed cases had an accuracy score of 70.56%, and daily active cases had an accuracy score of 72.22%.

8.7 MOVING AVERAGE

The moving average (MA) (spccharts online) is a simple analysis tool which smooths data by creating a consistent average over a specific period of time, like time, days or weeks. In a MA chart, the initial setup typically involves establishing UCL (Upper Control Limit), LCL (Lower Control Limit), and Target (Centerline) values. These limits are calculated based on monitoring and sampling the data when it is running while "in control". The formulas for MA charts are listed below.

Calculate the μ_0 value as the mean of the actual data values. Let $(X_1, X_2,..., X_N)$ be the measurement values of the N sample intervals. Or you can use a $\mu0$ value that you know from previous runs.

$$\mu_0 = \bar{X} = \left(\frac{1}{N} \sum_{i=1}^{N} X_i = \frac{(A_1 + A_2 + ... + A_N)}{N} \right)$$

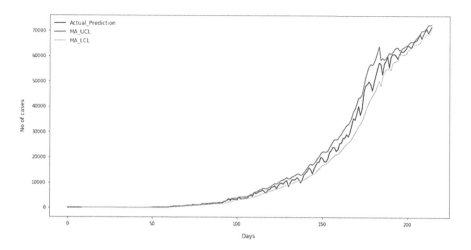

FIGURE 8.15 Graph shows the daily growth of confirmed cases in India from 30th January, 2020 to 31st July, 2020 and predicts the confirmed cases for next 30 days using Moving Average (MA).
Source: Data compiled by India Data (https://api.covid19india.org/csv/latest/state_wise_daily.csv), data as of 31th July, 2020

The standard deviation value (σ for the process is calculated using the sample standard deviation formula, seen below.

$$\sigma = \sqrt{\frac{\sum_{i=1}^{N} X_i - \bar{x}}{N-1}}$$

Assume the predict data by using the moving average (1 day per subinterval, 30 days intervals (N)). The MA upper and lower control limit can be calculated using the following formula. The target is predicted based on *randomrange()* function between upper control limit and lower control limit.

Control Limits for the MA chart

$$UCL = \mu_0 + 3*\frac{\sigma}{\sqrt{M}}$$

Target = randomrange (UCL, LCL)

$$LCL = \mu_0 - 3*\frac{\sigma}{\sqrt{M}}$$

Where
  μ_0 is the process mean
  σ is the process standard deviation, also known as sigma
  M is the length of the MA used to calculate the current value

TABLE 8.3

Prediction for daily confirmed, active and deceased SARS-CoV-2 (COVID-19) cases in India using MA and LSTM network model

	Moving Average				LSTM		
Days	Confirmed	Active	Deceased	Days	Confirmed	Active	Deceased
185	52,746	16,763	878	185	47,838	15,708	933
186	56,997	18,142	950	186	48,518	15,931	946
187	58,192	18,826	985	187	49,195	16,153	959
188	59,916	16,740	877	188	49,869	16,374	972
189	55,589	18,642	976	189	50,539	16,594	985
190	59,959	17,362	909	190	51,206	16,813	998
191	60,977	19,208	1005	191	51,870	17,031	1,011
192	60,921	18,296	958	192	52,530	17,248	1,024
193	60,407	19,178	1,003	193	53,187	17,463	1,037
194	59,088	19,448	1,017	194	53,839	17,677	1,049
195	60,778	18,969	993	195	54,488	17,890	1,062
196	62,211	19,704	1,031	196	55,134	18,102	1,074
197	61,779	19,293	1,009	197	55,775	18,313	1,087
198	62,441	19,922	1,042	198	56,412	18,522	1,099
199	63,171	20,203	1,057	199	57,045	18,730	1,112
200	64,414	19,710	1,031	200	57,674	18,936	1,124
201	63,905	19,890	1,040	201	58,299	19,141	1,136
202	63,382	20,260	1,060	202	58,920	19,345	1,148
203	65,088	20,283	1,061	203	59,536	19,547	1,160
204	66,035	20,439	1,069	204	60,148	19,748	1,172
205	66,334	20,896	1,093	205	60,756	19,947	1,184
206	67,382	21,037	1,100	206	61,360	20,146	1,195
207	68,918	21,434	1,121	207	61,960	20,343	1,207
208	67,045	21,696	1,135	208	62,555	20,538	1,218
209	68,708	21,279	1,113	209	63,146	20,732	1,230
210	69,862	22,098	1,155	210	63,733	20,924	1,241
211	70,897	21,922	1,146	211	64,315	21,115	1,253
212	69,222	22,110	1,156	212	64,893	21,305	1,264
213	70,481	22,193	1,160	213	65,468	21,494	1,275
214	71,654	22,598	1,181	214	66,038	21,681	1,286

8.8 RESULTS AND DISCUSSION

The LSTM network model and moving average (MA) techniques are used to predict the future 30 days (185th day to 214th day) from 1th August, 2020 to 30th August, 2020. In both techniques, predictions for daily confirmed, active and deceased SARS-CoV-2 (COVID-19) cases in India are listed in Table 8.3. Figure 8.15 shows the growth of daily confirmed cases with 30 days prediction of confirmed cases along with future 30 days prediction of confirmed cases in India using moving average (MA) techniques.

8.9 CONCLUSION

In this chapter, LSTM algorithm-based deep-learning models for confirmed, active and deceased cases in the state of India are developed for the spread of COVID-19 epidemic. Here we have considered the actual confirmed, active and deceased COVID-19 cases in the states of India. The numerical prediction for daily confirmed, active and deceased SARS-CoV-2 (COVID-19) cases in India using MA and LSTM network model for future 30 days, is well-adapted to the reported data and reflects the reality in India. The results proved a good concord between the reported data and the estimated data given by the proposed models. The forecast results show future tendency of COVID-19 spread in India and we strongly recommend that severe restrictions in containment zones and continuous health monitoring of suspected cases will cut down the local transmission and community spread.

REFERENCES

Allam, Zaheer, Dey Gourav, and David S. Jones. "Artificial intelligence (AI) provided early detection of the coronavirus (COVID-19) in China and will influence future Urban health policy internationally." *AI* 1, no. 2 (2020): 156–165.

Aroraa, Parul, Himanshu Kumarb, Bijaya Ketan Panigrahi. "Prediction and analysis of COVID-19positive cases using deep learning models: A descriptive case study of India". *Chaos, Solitons & Fractals*, 139, October 2020. https://doi.org/10.1016/j.chaos.2020.110017.

COVID-19, ICMR. COVID-19. Indian Council of Medical Research. Government of India. *ICMR* (2020). Available online at: https://www.icmr.gov.in/. Accessed July31st, 2020.

COVID-19Tracker India. https://www.covid19india.org/. Accessed July31st, 2020.

Gao, Yang, Jeff M. Phillips, Yan Zheng, Renqiang Min, P. Thomas Fletcher, and Guido Gerig. "Fully convolutional structured LSTM networks for joint 4D medical image segmentation." In *2018 IEEE 15th International Symposium on Biomedical Imaging (ISBI 2018)*, pp. 1104–1108. IEEE, 2018.

Litjens, Geert, Thijs Kooi, Babak Ehteshami Bejnordi, Arnaud Arindra Adiyoso Setio, Francesco Ciompi, Mohsen Ghafoorian, Jeroen Awm Van Der Laak, Bram Van Ginneken, and Clara I. Sánchez. "A survey on deep learning in medical image analysis." *Medical Image Analysis* 42 (2017): 60–88.

Liu, Feng, Zhigang Chen, and Jie Wang. "Video image target monitoring based on RNN-LSTM." *Multimedia Tools and Applications* 78, no. 4 (2019): 4527–4544.

MoHFW Home. https://www.mohfw.gov.in/. Accessed July31st, 2020.

Narin, Ali, Ceren Kaya, and Ziynet Pamuk. "Automatic detection of coronavirus disease (COVID-19) using x-ray images and deep convolutional neural networks." *arXiv preprint arXiv:2003.10849* (2020).

Punn, Narinder Singh, Sanjay Kumar Sonbhadra, and Sonali Agarwal. "COVID-19 epidemic analysis using machine learning and deep learning algorithms." *medRxiv* (2020). Available: https://www.medrxiv.org/content/early/2020/04/11/2020.04.08.20057679.

Qiu, Jiayu, Bin Wang, and Changjun Zhou. "Forecasting stock prices with long-short term memory neural network based on attention mechanism." *PloS one* 15, no. 1 (2020): e0227222.

Singh, Dilbag, Vijay Kumar, and Manjit Kaur. "Classification of COVID-19patients from chest CT images using multi-objective differential evolution–based convolutional neural networks." *European Journal of Clinical Microbiology & Infectious Diseases* 39, no. (2020): 1379–1389.

Toderici, George, Damien Vincent, Nick Johnston, Sung Jin Hwang, David Minnen, Joel Shor, and Michele Covell. "Full resolution image compression with recurrent neural networks." In *Proceedings of the IEEE Conference on Computer Vision and Pattern Recognition*, pp. 5306–5314. 2017.

Tomar, Anuradha, Neeraj Gupta, "Prediction for the spread of COVID-19in India and effectiveness of preventive measures". *Science of The Total Environment* 728, 1 August (2020).

Index